THE Esquire GUIDE TO BODYWEIGHT TRAINING

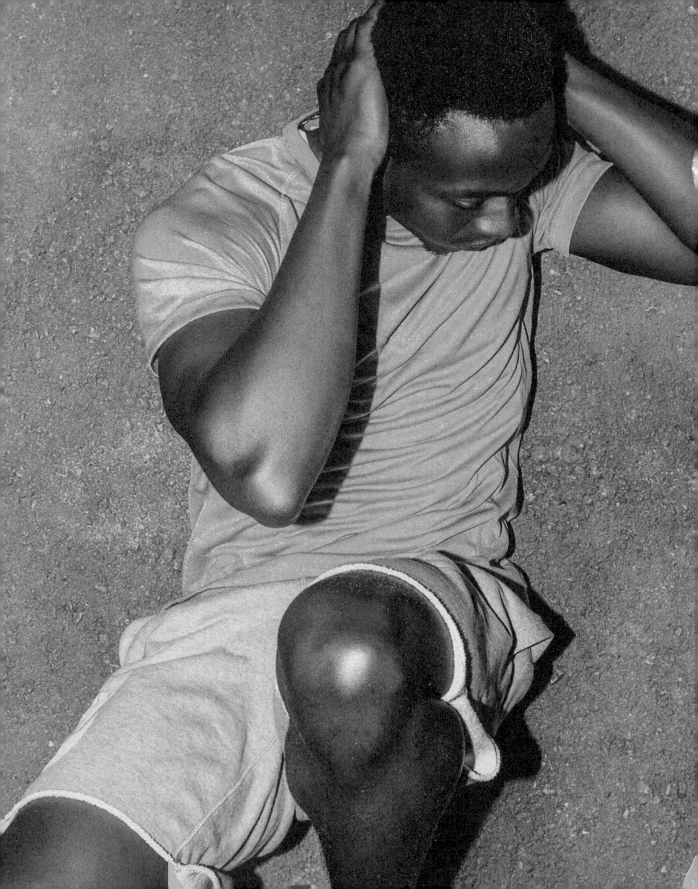

THE *Esquire*
GUIDE TO
BODYWEIGHT TRAINING

CALISTHENICS TO LOOK AND FEEL YOUR BEST
FROM THE BOARDROOM TO THE BEDROOM

ADAM SCHERSTEN WITH CHRIS KLIMEK

ROCKRIDGE
PRESS

For general information on our other products and services or to obtain technical support, please contact our Customer Care Department within the United States at (866) 744-2665, or outside the United States at (510) 253-0500.

Rockridge Press publishes its books in a variety of electronic and print formats. Some content that appears in print may not be available in electronic books, and vice versa.

TRADEMARKS: Rockridge Press and the Rockridge Press logo are trademarks or registered trademarks of Callisto Media Inc. and/or its affiliates, in the United States and other countries, and may not be used without written permission. All other trademarks are the property of their respective owners. Rockridge Press is not associated with any product or vendor mentioned in this book.

FRONT COVER PHOTO: PeopleImages.com/Getty
BACK COVER PHOTO: Studio Firma/Stocksy
AUTHOR PHOTO: Philip Bell

INTERIOR PHOTOS: Studio Firma/Stocksy, pg. 2; BONNINSTUDIO/Stocksy, pg. 6; BONNINSTUDIO/Stocksy, pg. 12; AP, pg. 21; MOSUNO/Stocksy, pg. 22; Rob & Julia Campbell/Stocksy, pg. 84; Image Source/Alamy, pg. 126; BONNINSTUDIO/Stocksy, pg. 160; Cultura Creative/Alamy, pg. 202; Jovana Rikalo/Stocksy, pg. 244. All other photos Shutterstock.com

ILLUSTRATIONS © Christian Papazoglakis

ISBN: Print 978-1-62315-702-9 | eBook 978-1-62315-703-6

TO MY CLIENTS,
FOR ALWAYS KEEPING ME
ON MY TOES

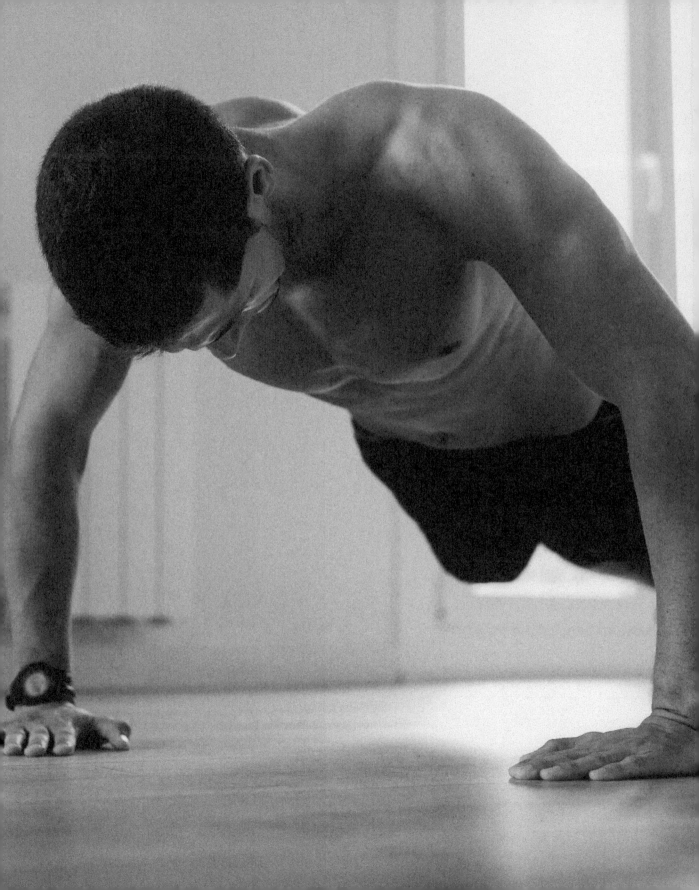

CONTENTS

RAW STRENGTH

Facts of the Fittest

The US Army requires that men who are between 22 and 26 years old be able to

RUN TWO MILES
IN 16:30
and do
40 PUSH-UPS
and
50 SIT-UPS
—each in less than 2 minutes

. . . .

ANGUS MACASKILL, THE STRONGEST MAN OF ALL TIME,

was 7 foot 4 inches tall, weighed roughly 500 pounds, and purportedly could lift a 2,800-pound ship's anchor to his chest

Martial artist and actor
BRUCE LEE
was known to perform push-ups
USING JUST
TWO FINGERS

. . . .

Ashrita Furman, who holds 121 Guinness World Record titles— the most of all time— first made his mark on the records community by doing

27,000
CONSECUTIVE JUMPING JACKS
in 1979

. . . .

The average man can perform between 1 and 12 chin-ups with good form.

GUY
SCHOTT,
THE GUINNESS WORLD
RECORD HOLDER,
CAN DO 57—
IN ONE MINUTE

FOREWORD

Esquire was founded in 1933 with a simple mission: to help men live better and more enriching lives. For over eighty years we've done this by focusing on the essentials, the little—and sometimes big—things that a man needs to know in order to better navigate the world. How to make the perfect Manhattan. How tie a Windsor knot. How to buy a tuxedo. The classics are classic for a reason—because they work and they've stood the test of time. Like the push-up, the crunch, the squat.

For the last eight years or so, my own exercise regimen has consisted of a combination of bodyweight exercises, cardiovascular torture, isometrics, and kettle bells. Most of this is basic stuff, easily replicable for me no matter where I happen to be, from home alone to on the road in some underequipped hotel fitness center. Now, I'm no paragon of fitness. I enjoy my life—sometimes a lot. But my regimen has enabled me to continue competing at a relatively high level. I still sometimes run the golf course rather than use a cart. I still can be a force from the other side of the tennis net.

Fads, whether in fashion, food, or fitness, are as transient as the latest Katy Perry song or viral video. But the fundamentals remain, the building blocks of a well-lived life.

We at *Esquire* would know. Back in February 1950, we published a series of articles called "The Art of Keeping Fit" that offered the fitness routines of ten notable men such as FBI chief J. Edgar Hoover, author James A. Michener, and Henry Ford II—along with a guide to lunges, leg lifts, and using chairs for elevated push-ups. "Half-hearted waving of weights should be left to the dumbbells," we wrote. Instead, we suggested calisthenics to strengthen the full body. Our championing of this do-anywhere approach to exercise has never wavered, whether in our Ultimate Fitness Guides of the mid-1980s, our Better Man service sections of the mid-aughts, or today, as *Esquire* embarks on a national fitness challenge with partners Equinox and the Mayo Clinic built around calisthenics and many of the exercises that appear in this book.

Along with fundamental bodyweight exercises, we've also based our health advice on eating smart and eating well. No crazy meat-only, fruit-only, juice-only diets that put your body through short-term misery for elusive results. Instead, we suggest moderation (mixed with the occasional steak and tequila) and common sense. Exercise legend Jack LaLanne put it best when he offered up this gem in a 2004 interview for our "What I've Learned" column: "Would you get your dog up every day, give him a cup of coffee, a doughnut, and a cigarette? Hell no, you'd kill the damn dog."

Like Jack himself was, this book is no bullshit. It's simple and clear and if you make even a reasonable attempt at Adam Schersten's bodyweight training programs, the benefits will be considerable.

DAVID GRANGER
Editor in Chief, *Esquire*

INTRODUCTION

In 2007, I left the States for a remote island off the coast of Honduras. It wasn't exactly a career move. At the time, all I wanted to do was teach scuba diving and put off getting a desk job. I'd been a fitness fanatic for years before hopping on the plane and landing in the middle of nowhere, so I felt anxious when it dawned on me that I'd have virtually no access to traditional gym equipment. After a little research, I realized that calisthenics was my best option (my only one, really) for staying in shape. It was then that I put together my first bodyweight circuits.

For the next four years, I traveled to various parts of Central America, integrating my circuits wherever and whenever I could. When I found I was able to maintain strength and size, and even build my endurance, I understood the raw power of calisthenics.

Being strong is more than being able to bench press or squat 300 pounds. It's about keeping every part of your body fit while allowing your joints to work through a full range of motion. The exercises and workout programs outlined in this book will get you ready for everything, from a grueling backpacking trip to helping a friend move out of a fifth-floor walk-up to simply taking off your shirt at the beach with confidence. You'll learn how to get strong, stay (or get) slim, and decrease your risk of injury.

The word *calisthenics* comes from the Greek words *kallos*, meaning "beauty," and *sthenos*, meaning "strength." Calisthenic exercises work to develop a lean, muscular, statuesque body—a body to be admired, like a work of art. Whether you're totally new to regular exercise or have been weight training for years, the innovative techniques and customizable workouts in this book will make peak physical fitness your reality— while changing your perspective on what it means to be strong. Let's get started.

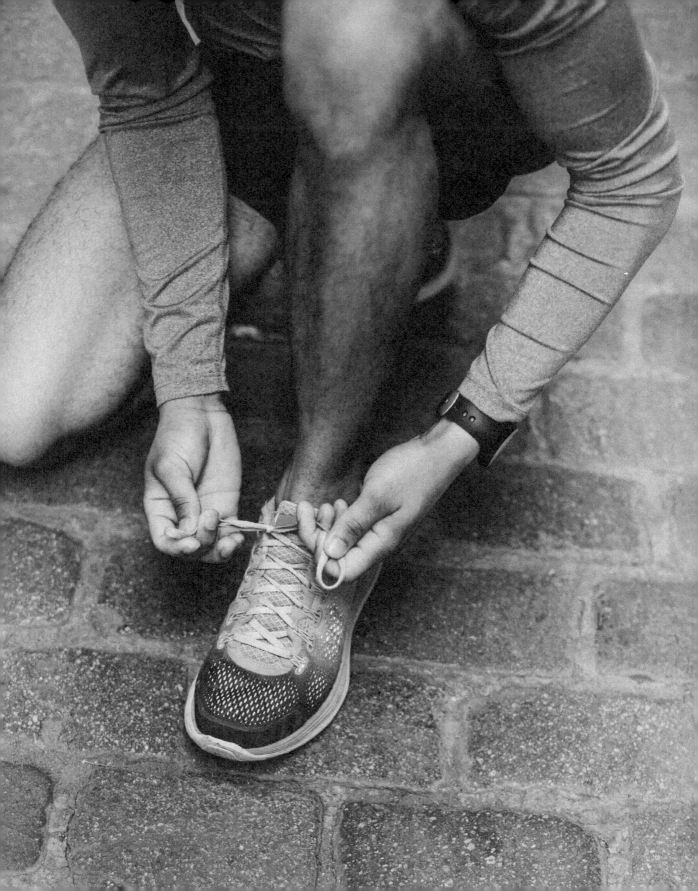

ONE

According to the American College of Sports Medicine's worldwide survey of fitness trends, bodyweight training was the top fitness trend of 2015—but it's nothing new to the fitness world. Bodyweight training is just another word for training that consists of calisthenics exercises; that is, exercises that use your own body's weight to create resistance and build muscle.

FIT FOR ANYTHING

No bench press. No dumbbells. No sweaty guy grunting through his WOD next to you. Just a set of rigorous, do-anywhere exercises that will chisel every part of your body. By focusing on movements—such as pushes and pulls—that target several muscle groups simultaneously, as opposed to working one muscle group at a time, bodyweight exercises make it possible to do a balanced 30-minute workout that challenges the arms, chest, core, and legs.

THE BODYWEIGHT BENEFITS

Bodyweight training or calisthenics—the two terms are used here more or less interchangeably—is experiencing a resurgence because it's easy to incorporate into any schedule and it gets results. It can be done in conjunction with other weight and cardio programs, or it can be a stand-alone approach. You can easily modify it as your fitness level improves, and you don't need any added weights or machines. More specifically, here are some key reasons why I use it with my clients.

FULL-BODY WORKOUT

Because bodyweight training works several muscle groups, rather than one in isolation, it delivers results in less time than other fitness techniques. By doing quick bodyweight cardio moves like burpees or jumping jacks in between strength moves like push-ups and pull-ups, you get strength training, cardio exercise, and core work all in the same exercise routine. The shorter rest times that often accompany bodyweight training help you maintain a higher heart rate, which increases cardiovascular capacity and helps to create lean muscle mass.

EXERCISE ANYWHERE

Bodyweight training can be done anywhere, so it's perfect for the busy executive, the frequent traveler, or anyone who hates the scene at the health club. One of my favorite places to do a calisthenics routine is outdoors—on the beach, at a park, or even at a playground where I can incorporate the jungle gym into my routine. Getting out in nature also has the added bonus of relaxing your mind. When I travel, it doesn't matter to me if the hotel has a treadmill or set of weight machines as long as there is enough space in my room or somewhere outside for me to knock out a calisthenics workout.

ONE EXERCISE, MANY VARIATIONS

Machines have a limited ability to adapt to your level of fitness, but you can customize bodyweight training to you, regardless of whether you're a total beginner or an incredibly fit person looking for your next challenge. A push-up, for example, has many levels of difficulty. You can progress from doing it on your knees to your feet, add a stability challenge, or make it dynamic by adding movement. Other ways to tailor the routine to your fitness level include adding repetitions, performing the move superfast or very slowly, and varying your rest time. Playing with these variations will help keep you from getting bored of doing the same routine day in and day out.

WHAT I'VE LEARNED

I wasn't real quick, and I wasn't real strong. Some guys will just take off and it's like, whoa. So I beat them with my mind and my fundamentals.
—LARRY BIRD

REAL-WORLD FIT

Bodyweight exercises teach you how to maneuver your body in the real world, not just on a leg press machine. When you work out with weights, you can get stuck training muscles with limited movement patterns. You lie on a bench or sit on a machine at the gym, engaging your arms or legs but letting your core sit idle. While you may have an impressive deadlift, go out on the tennis court for an hour, and you'll be incredibly sore the next day. Why? Because even though your muscles are strong, they're not used to any movements except the ones you make at the gym. To perform real-world movements, your body must provide real-world stability—and calisthenics never allows for an idle core.

INJURY PREVENTION

Working out is supposed to build a body that's harder to injure, not easier. Yet gym-related injuries, particularly during weight training, are common. In many weight-lifting programs, people overwork some muscles and underwork others. This leads to muscle imbalances, which leave joints susceptible to injury. Because bodyweight training works the whole body all the time, your muscles get strong as a complete system, moving and stabilizing in concert. This is particularly important when you think about the core stabilizers that protect your most precious commodity: the spine.

It's important to add that injury isn't something that only happens at the gym; it can happen with calisthenics as well. Many people begin a fitness program with

FORE!

BODYWEIGHT TRAINING FOR THE BEST GOLF OF YOUR LIFE

> Bodyweight training will make you feel and look better. As an added bonus, it'll also improve your golf game.

"You can unlock a lot of power in the golf swing if you're more mobile," says Andrew Losik. He would know: He spent five years as a PGA professional before becoming a certified personal trainer at AXIS Personal Trainers in Menlo Park, California. "The golf swing is a 100 percent maximal effort movement, like jumping up on something really high."

The way to nail that swing while protecting your lower back from injury is to strengthen your glutes and your core—the king and queen of the golf swing, as they're called—which will let you nail the finer technical points of the swing. "If you're right-handed, you want to transfer your weight to your left side through the swing," Losik says. "A lot of guys don't do that."

For golfers just getting started with bodyweight exercises, Losik recommends a circuit of three sets of exercises that target the chain of muscles needed to swing a club with accuracy and power.

Set 1: 20 squats and 20 oblique crunches, followed by lunges—walking, backward, and side, 5 per leg in each direction.

Set 2: Push-ups with a reach for the ceiling at the top of the move, alternating sides, 10 reps on each.

Set 3: Two 30-second planks on the elbows, keeping the abs squeezed and the back straight.

Repeat the whole circuit three or four times. Once you've built a solid foundation, see MyTPI.com for more specific techniques to help your swing.

preexisting injuries, muscle imbalances, and reduced mobility. It's crucial to be aware of and address these issues before starting a bodyweight training program. If you're unsure of your readiness for the exercises and workouts in this book, first seek the advice of a trusted personal trainer or physical therapist.

A STRONG BODY BEGINS WITH MOBILITY

We are all mobile to a certain degree, due in part to our genetics and in part to the movements (or lack of movement) our bodies go through daily. If you spend 8 to 10 hours a day sitting at your desk, and then a couple of hours in front of the television at night, there's no getting around the fact that your mobility will suffer. And if your body can't comfortably get into a certain position because of a mobility restriction, no amount of strength training will fix that. Start paying close attention to your movements and begin to identify your physical limitations. By focusing on mobility, you'll improve your body's functionality and flexibility, as well as what you're probably most interested in: strength.

If your focus is on building strength and you're skimming this section, remember this: If a muscle can't achieve its ideal length, it will never achieve its ideal strength. Consider the squat. If you perform a squat with your hips in the correct position, your

quads, glutes, and hamstrings do most of the work, supported by your calves, hip stabilizers, and core. This makes your upper legs muscular and strong. But let's say your mobility is low. Maybe your calves are tight. When you go to do a squat, the foreshortened muscles won't allow your center of gravity to shift forward enough. To avoid falling backward, you'll have to lean far forward, putting stress on your lower back. Not only will you risk injury, you'll prevent your thighs and glutes from building necessary strength to execute the move.

For maximum effect, it's best to do your mobility work after your body is warm and your muscles are malleable, which is why you should always incorporate it into the cooldown section of every workout. I challenge you to hold your stretches for one to two minutes at a time, allowing your muscles time to cool in an elongated position. You'll be surprised at how much you can improve your range of motion over time. This book includes a set of mobility exercises for you to choose from (see page 257) after your workouts.

PUSH (AND PULL) YOUR LIMITS

If you're used to going to the gym for chest days or leg days, it's time to change the way you think about exercise. Because my bodyweight routines are total-body workouts, the way I've grouped exercises is different. Bodyweight exercises don't focus on which individual muscles you're targeting, because each movement uses numerous big and small muscles throughout the body. Instead, they focus on the primary movement your body makes. I've divided these movements into five categories: push, pull, hip-driven, ankle-driven, and core exercises.

PUSH

One of the main multijoint actions of the upper body is pushing, whether it's from a horizontal position, as in a classic push-up, or from a vertical one, as in a pike push-up or dip. Pushing movements primarily target the chest (pectorals), shoulders (deltoids), and triceps.

PULL

The other major multijoint movement of the upper body is pulling. Like pushing, pulling can be done horizontally, as in a row, or vertically, as in a pull-up or chin-up. These exercises focus primarily on the trapezius, rhomboid, latissimus dorsi (lats), and biceps muscles.

HIP-DRIVEN

These movements originate in the hips, glutes, and thighs, with minimal motion from the ankle and none from the lower back. The primary muscles worked most in hip-driven exercises are the glutes and hamstrings. Examples of hip-driven exercises are hip hinges and bridges.

ANKLE-DRIVEN

Ankle-driven movements require bending at the ankle, in a process called dorsiflexion, which happens when the shin is allowed to move forward over the center of the foot. These exercises call for the ankle, knee, and hip to move as one unit, and they target the quads, glutes, hamstrings, calves, and hip flexors. Examples include squats, lunges, and jumps. Most people have tight calves, which should be addressed before these moves can be done correctly. Be sure to stretch your calves if you feel your feet turning out during these exercises.

LOW BACK IN BLACK

> If simply lifting your kid, or standing up from your desk, sends a ripple of pain through your lower back, you're not alone: The University of Maryland Medical Center says that 60 to 80 percent of adults in the U.S. live with occasional lower-back pain. White-collar warriors are especially vulnerable, because spending upward of eight hours a day sitting shortens your hamstrings and hip flexors and reduces overall hip mobility.

Prolonged sitting can be damaging even if you're conscientious about exercise, so when you're at the office, stand up and stroll over to the water cooler or the window on the far side of the floor at least once per hour—even if you went jogging before you hit the office or you're playing pickup basketball after work. If you manage a few simple stretches in your cubicle or hotel room, all the better. Leaving a few minutes at the end of your workout to perform a few stretches for the hips is the best way to ensure that infrequent, mild lower-back pain doesn't spiral into chronic agony.

CORE

In order to do any exercises in the four other categories, you're going to need a solid core so that your limbs will have a stable platform from which to push, pull, or otherwise gain leverage. The core provides this stability by controlling pelvic tilt and preventing excessive flexion, extension, or rotation from the spine. The muscles that make up the core are numerous, but for simplicity we'll focus on the abdominals (rectus abdominis) and internal and external obliques. The hip muscles as well as the spinal erectors and several other back muscles are also core muscles but will be worked on in other categories. To target the core, you'll use movements like planks, crunches, and crawls.

WHAT YOU'LL NEED

While you can get a total bodyweight workout without using any extra equipment, if you have a few items on hand, you can significantly expand the number of exercises available to you and keep your body and mind from getting bored. Here are a few things I recommend:

FOAM ROLLER A foam roller is a great pre- and postworkout tool for warming up muscles and breaking apart adhesions. It's not quite as good as a real massage, but it's not a bad alternative.

PULL-UP BAR Having a simple bar at home makes it easy to do basic pull-ups and chin-ups in addition to knee raises, negative pull-ups, and more.

GIVE 'EM ENOUGH ROPE

> A good jump rope is one of the most economical and portable pieces of fitness equipment you can buy. A high-quality plastic speed rope costs $10 or $12 and takes up less space in your suitcase or gym bag than your running shoes. Performed at maximal effort, jumping rope is a taxing cardio workout all on its own; at a more relaxed pace, it's a great warm-up for almost any sort of high-intensity athletic activity—and it's a lifesaver for treadmill-averse travelers. For a successful jump-rope session, a few tips:

- Make sure you're using a rope appropriate to your height. If you step on the rope's midpoint, each handle should come up to your armpits.
- Avoid grass and use a solid surface for jumping, like the parking lot at your office or hotel.
- To maintain good form, keep your elbows in by your ribs, flick the rope with your wrists, and don't waste energy jumping higher than necessary to clear the rope—a couple inches will do.

Once you can reliably sustain one skip per second for three minutes, you can try some of the fancier stuff you've seen in boxing movies.

STEP This can be as simple as a step stool or the bottom step of a staircase. The step will add a cardio element to exercises, allow you to do moves on an incline or decline, and add variation on lunges.

TRX This compact, lightweight tool can turn your home, hotel room, or nearby outdoor space into a calisthenics playground. It instantly gives you something to row from and has the potential for countless exercise variations.

MUSCLE GROUP ANATOMY

A VISUAL REFERENCE

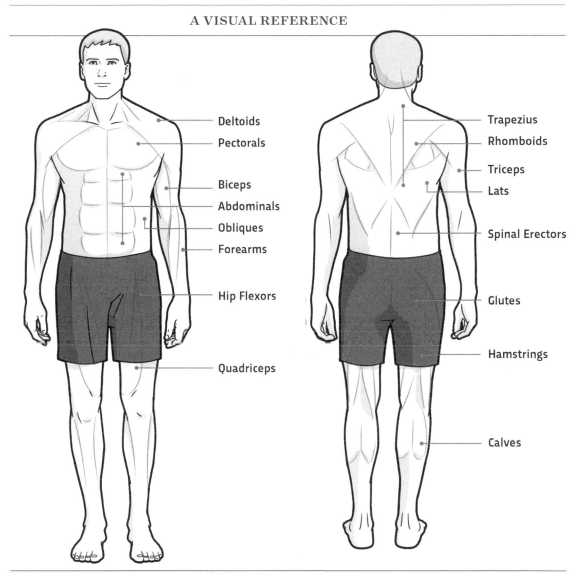

Deltoids
Pectorals
Biceps
Abdominals
Obliques
Forearms
Hip Flexors
Quadriceps

Trapezius
Rhomboids
Triceps
Lats
Spinal Erectors
Glutes
Hamstrings
Calves

MOVEMENTS TARGETED BY MUSCLE GROUP:	CORE	ANKLE DRIVEN	HIP DRIVEN	PUSH	PULL
	Abdominals	Calves	Glutes	Deltoids	Biceps
	Obliques	Glutes	Hamstrings	Pectorals	Lats
		Hamstrings		Triceps	Trapezius
		Quadriceps			

Pick one day per month to test yourself. How many flawless squats can you knock out in 60 seconds? How many arms-locked push-ups? Only the ones you execute with perfect form count. Try to raise your total by five from whatever it was last month.

MONKEY AROUND

> For a lot of guys, particularly those of us who love the outdoors, the worst part of the gym is *the gym*. An outdoor playground can be a great substitute when you're on the road, or just a fun place to change up your regimen—especially if you run there and run home.

See those monkey bars? I don't—I see a pull-up bar. For adult-size grip spacing, you'll probably have to use the thicker support bars on either side of the apparatus instead of the ones the kiddies cling to, which will challenge your grip strength. Or you can use the monkey bars as intended—that is, to hang—for a great active rest. You'll probably also have to curl your heels back so your feet don't touch the ground while doing pull-ups. For an extra challenge, tuck your knees into your chest or stick both legs horizontally in front of you, holding your body in an L-shape while doing them.

Playgrounds also offer lots of surfaces you can use to prop up your feet while performing step-ups, plank walk-ups, and other activities that need elevation. And because their designs vary so substantially, you'll be forced to get creative.

PROGRESSION AND REGRESSION

Don't be fooled into thinking that calisthenics exercises are a regression from lifting weights. Technically, a push-up is a progression from the bench press. Sure, you can add more weight to the bench press to increase the challenge, but that movement is actually easier for the body because it doesn't have the stability component the push-up has. Within calisthenics exercises, you can—and will—progress, too. Once you've perfected the standard push-up, you can increase the difficulty by moving your hands closer together or tapping your shoulders between reps. But at the start, your focus should be on perfect form, not progression. If you can't yet do a proper push-up, recognize the value of a regression, starting from your knees or, preferably, from an elevated surface. Don't skip the building blocks. Once you perfect your form, you can move on to a full push-up.

In each of the exercise chapters, you'll find groups of three exercises. The first exercise of each group is always a basic version for you to master before moving on to the progressions that follow it. The progressions take the basic exercise to a new challenge. Sometimes they build on each other, and sometimes they go in different directions of difficulty. Either way, form should be mastered before moving on. If you're having trouble with the basic version, simplify it. Some exercises will have tips to help you do just that.

JACK LALANNE
1914–2011

Interviewed in 2004 by CAL FUSSMAN

I'm going to be ninety in September. Everybody else can have a piece of the birthday cake, but not me. I have rules, and I follow 'em. No cake, no pie, no candy, no ice cream! Haven't had any in seventy-five years. It makes me feel great not eating birthday cake. That's the gift I give myself.

Forget about what you used to do. This is the moment you've been waiting for.

As long as the emphasis is on winning, you're gonna have steroids.

If man makes it, don't eat it.

You've got to satisfy you. If you can't satisfy you, you're a failure.

I work out for two hours every morning, seven days a week—even when I'm traveling. I hate it. But I love the result! That's the key, baby!

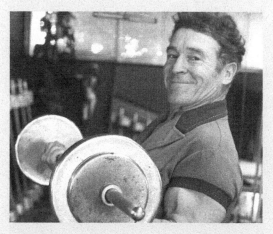

Fitness guru Jack LaLanne pumps iron in his home in Hollywood, California, 1980

If you want to change somebody, don't preach to him. Set an example and shut up.

Scales lie! You lose thirty pounds of muscle and you gain thirty pounds of fat and you weigh the same, right? Take that tape measure out. That won't lie. Your waistline is your lifeline. It should be the same as it was when you were a young person.

Sex is giving, giving, giving. The more energy you have, the more you're going to please.

The guy who's most impressed me is Paul C. Bragg. He completely saved my life. When I was a kid, I was addicted to sugar. I was a skinny kid with pimples. Used to eat ice cream by the quart. I had blinding headaches. I tried to commit suicide. And then one day, my life changed. Bragg was a nutritionist. My mother and I were a little late getting to his lecture. The place was packed, and so we started to leave. But Bragg said, "We don't turn anybody away here. Ushers, bring two seats. Put those two up on the stage." It was the most humiliating moment. There I was, up on stage. I was so ashamed of the way I looked, I didn't want people to see me. Little did I know they had problems, too. And Bragg said, "It doesn't matter what your age is, what your physical condition is. If you obey nature's laws, you can be born again." From that moment on, I completely changed my diet, began to exercise, and went on to become captain of the football team. And do you know something? Every time I get ready to lecture, I think, If I can just help one person like I was helped . . .

Would you get your dog up every day, give him a cup of coffee, a doughnut, and a cigarette? Hell, no. You'd kill the damn dog.

Go on, have a glass of wine with dinner. What is wine, anyway? Pure grapes. A glass of wine is much better for you than a Coke.

What I do isn't about money. Can you put a price on a human life?

I can't afford to die. It'll wreck my image.

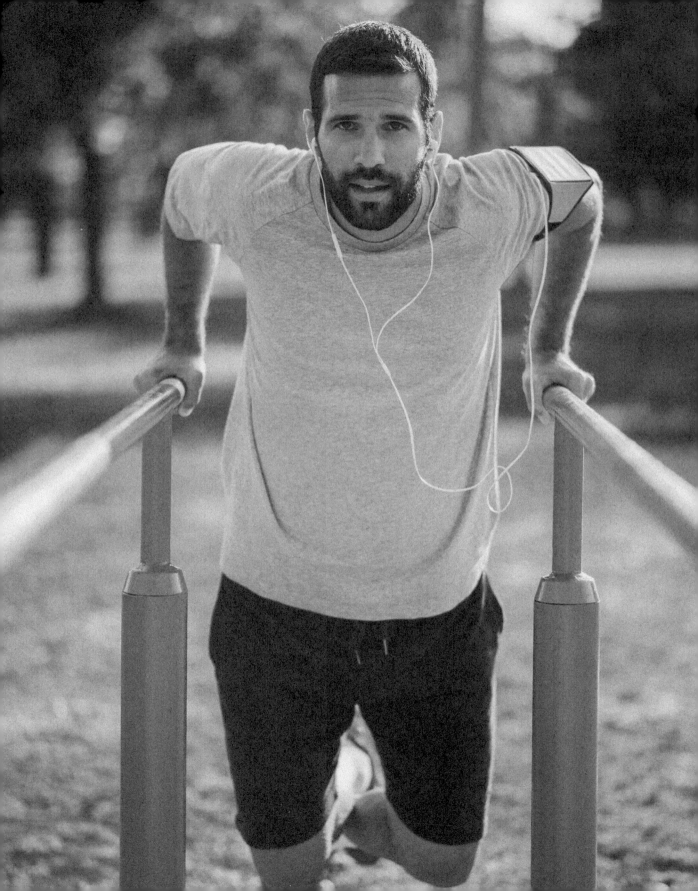

TWO

No matter how often or how hard you work out, if you eat poorly, or not enough, you'll never get the results you want. You can't work like a horse and eat like a chicken and expect to gain muscle. Your muscles need protein and carbs, and lots of them, to build new tissue. In this section, I dive into the necessary nutritional information—just enough but no more—that'll help

FUEL & GEAR

you eat right for your fitness goals. Toward the end I offer a quick overview of the best things to wear for a bodyweight workout, from shirt to shoes to headphones. And don't miss the playlist at the end of the chapter to get you moving and grooving.

Deciding what to eat shouldn't be complicated. Here are four simple principles to keep in mind.

PRINCIPLE 1: EAT REAL FOOD

Walk through the typical American grocery store and read the labels on the food. With all the synthetic chemicals and processed ingredients, much of what's on the shelf barely counts as food at all. Our bodies didn't evolve to live on potato chips, soda, and frozen meals. I follow author Michael Pollan's advice to eat real food. Buy ingredients—fresh produce, meats, and dairy—instead of processed, pre-prepared foods. If you buy organic, you can be sure your produce and grains haven't been treated with pesticides.

PRINCIPLE 2: EAT WHAT YOU NEED

According to the National Institutes of Health, meals in restaurants have grown twice or even three times as big as they were 20 years ago, and obesity rates have kept pace. In 1971, 14.1 percent of Americans were obese. Today it's 34.9 percent, and supersized meals are a major reason why.

Many Americans don't realize it, but a serving of chicken should be the size of your palm, a bowl of cereal should be the size of your fist, and pasta should be limited to one handful per serving. When you eat what you need and combine that with a strategic workout plan, great results are inevitable.

PRINCIPLE 3: EAT MORE OFTEN

The idea of three meals a day is a throwback to a different era. If you're trying to gain muscle, three meals a day isn't going to cut it. If you're trying to lose body fat, it's better to eat smaller meals more frequently, about every 2 to 3 hours. Eating like this maintains your blood sugar at stable levels throughout the day and keeps your digestive system working. It also prevents that sluggish feeling we get when we eat too much, which I know completely kills my motivation to work out.

PRINCIPLE 4: FOOD TIMING

When you eat is just as important to achieving your fitness goals as what you eat. To build muscle, eat both carbs and protein before you exercise to get the energy you need to perform your best. Do the same thing after a workout, too. Many people emphasize eating just protein after exercise, but at that point, your body's main priority is refueling its glycogen stores. If all you eat postworkout is protein, your liver will break a large portion of that protein down and rebuild it as glucose to refill those stores, and only whatever's left over will be used to synthesize new muscle tissue. If you eat "protein-sparing" carbs postworkout, your body will use those carbs to refuel your glycogen stores, and all the protein you consume will be available for growth.

If you're trying to build muscle and get rid of fat, you want to eat a small amount of good fats before you work out. The idea is that if you consume, say, a handful of nuts, your body is already in a fat-processing mode when you start to work out, and you can keep that going as you exercise. If you're craving carbs after your workout, you have a two-hour window to eat them. Your metabolism is at its peak and your muscles are trying to replenish their exhausted glycogen stores, so your body will use those carbs for that instead of storing them as fat.

THE SPECIFICS

The key to smart eating for strengthening is to understand some basic information on how protein, carbohydrates, and fats, plus water, interact with each other and with your body. Fruit and pasta are both mainly carbs, for example, but your body processes them differently. The quality of each nutrient matters as much as the quantity.

PROTEIN

Proteins are made of building blocks called amino acids, which can be linked together in thousands of combinations to form different proteins. Most amino acids are made by the body, but eight of them are not and must come from food. These eight are known as the "essential amino acids." Animal products like dairy, eggs, and meat are called "complete proteins" because they contain all of the essential amino acids. Proteins that you find in foods such as beans and legumes are not complete because they may only have four or five of the essential amino acids—but, if eaten in the right combination with other foods, they can supply you with complete proteins. Your body doesn't store

THREE
PREWORKOUT
SNACKS

FOR MUSCLE GAIN

Whey protein shake

½ cup oatmeal

Banana

FOR BURNING FAT

Greek yogurt

Nuts

Berries

THREE
POSTWORKOUT
SNACKS

FOR MUSCLE GAIN

Peanut butter on rice cakes

Tuna on whole-wheat bread

Turkey and cheese with apple slices

FOR BURNING FAT

Hard-boiled egg and snap peas

Steamed vegetables and tofu

**Cottage cheese with blueberries
and whole-wheat toast**

protein like it does fat and carbs, so you need to eat it every day. Essential amino acids are key to growth, which is why it's critical that you consume enough complete proteins. If you're hoping to gain muscle, you should consume more than the baseline of 0.5 grams of complete protein per pound of body weight each day. Your daily goal should be to consume from 0.7 to 1 gram per pound of body weight.

CARBOHYDRATES

In recent years, carbs have gotten a bad rap, but just like protein, they're essential for an optimally functioning body. They supply nearly half of the energy you need, and certain carbs, like fiber, are necessary for digestion and toxin elimination. The trouble comes when we combine carbohydrate consumption with inactivity. The body converts both simple and complex carbs into glucose (sugar) for energy, but when we sit around for most of the day, those sugars circulate in the bloodstream instead of being used, eventually getting stored for the long term as fat.

If your main goal is to build muscle, I recommend that 55 to 60 percent of your calories come from carbs. If you're more focused on losing body fat, shoot for something closer to 45 percent, but remember that if you cut too many carbs out, you risk undermining your strength. Either way, choose complex carbs over simple ones, as it takes the body longer to digest complex carbs, resulting in less glucose available to turn into fat. You'll find complex carbs in whole foods like vegetables, nuts, beans, and whole grains.

A study published in the *American Journal of Clinical Nutrition* concluded that men consume more fat, sodium, and calories on days when they drink, even in moderation, than on days when they abstain.

FATS

Fats have been blamed for making us obese and causing cardiovascular disease, but this is not exactly the case. Fat in your diet is different from fat on your body. Fat is essential in order for your body to function properly.

An active person does not need to be afraid of eating fat, as it's a great source of energy. Roughly 30 percent of your daily caloric intake should come from fats. Believe it or not, if you're trying to lose fat and are exercising regularly, shoot for closer to 40 percent.

Be aware that fats come in two broad categories: saturated and unsaturated. Saturated fats are solid at room temperature—like butter, lard, or coconut oil. Unsaturated fats are liquid at room temperature—think olive oil, fish oil, or peanut oil. As you choose your fats, try to balance saturated with unsaturated.

BETTER, NOT LESS

FOODS FOR AN ACTIVE LIFESTYLE

Jennifer Koslo, an Austin, Texas–based nutritionist and board-certified sports dietitian who has competed in marathons and triathlons for decades, says that if you're looking to shed fat, pack on muscle, or both, the formula is simple: Adopt a consistent exercise routine, and create a moderate calorie deficit. "The key is to provide your body with the right balance of nutrients at the right time, and avoid extreme dips in calorie intake," she says. Overreliance on protein bars and shakes is a recipe for trouble; they're calorie bombs and can be high in unhealthy fats.

Trendy diets that eliminate entire food groups tend to produce only short-term results. Healthy snacks are essential to sustaining energy throughout the day and prevent overindulging in the really damaging stuff. Here are six that earn her approval:

- Hummus and veggies
- Nuts (1 ounce) and a piece of fruit
- Shelled edamame
- A slice of whole-grain bread with nut butter
- Oatmeal with sliced almonds and berries
- Beans wrapped in lettuce or a whole-grain tortilla

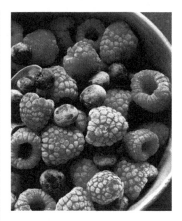

Koslo advises eating a variety of high-quality foods in moderation.

1 Stock up on frozen fruits and vegetables, which can be quickly mixed into smoothies and steamed, respectively.

2 Spend a few hours on the weekend cooking for the week ahead. Cook up some brown rice, grill a few chicken breasts, chop vegetables, and then store them in the refrigerator as individual servings.

3 Veggies add color and nutrient value to everything. Put spinach in your smoothies, cauliflower in your eggs, and butternut squash in your macaroni and cheese.

Ever been told that energy drinks and sports gels are a must when you're working out regularly? Koslo recommends skipping them. Most energy drinks are spiked with caffeine and sugar, and the way they disrupt your sleep will cancel out any modest performance enhancement they give you. And while sports gels do deliver the necessary sugar for training, they're also full of preservatives. Better to get the kick you need from raisins, dates, and other dried fruits.

PROTEIN BARS

SKIP THE STORE AND MAKE YOUR OWN

Most Americans are sedentary and tend to get more protein than they need. Unless you've just been cast in the next *Terminator* movie, odds are you're not looking to pack on pounds and pounds of muscle. You're probably aiming to get generally stronger and fitter so that more of your body weight is lean tissue rather than fat.

Protein bars deliver extra protein, but even the better ones usually also deliver calories, sugar, and sodium. If you're hooked on these bars, they're easy and much healthier to make yourself. Here's a simple recipe for a homemade bar you can make in less than 5 minutes from start to finish. Egg whites provide high-quality protein and act as a binder for energizing oats and antioxidant-rich cranberries, and flaxseed delivers healthy fats.

On days when you're feeling super lazy, just head for a jar of peanut butter. A two-tablespoon serving delivers 8 grams of protein. But make sure the only ingredients are peanuts and oil—and pass if you see sugar or hydrogenated oils in the ingredients list.

OATMEAL-CRANBERRY PROTEIN BAR

MAKES 1

¼ cup oats

1 teaspoon honey

1 tablespoon all-purpose flour

1 egg white

¼ teaspoon vanilla extract

¼ teaspoon baking powder

1 teaspoon ground cinnamon

1 tablespoon dried cranberries

2 tablespoons ground flaxseed

1 In a microwave-safe bowl or mug, mix the oats, honey, flour, egg white, vanilla, baking powder, cinnamon, cranberries, and flaxseed.

2 Flatten the mixture into the bottom of the bowl, and microwave on high for 45 seconds.

3 Once it's cool, pop the mixture out of the bowl and enjoy, or throw it into a zip-top bag and take it with you for later.

PER SERVING
CALORIES: 280
TOTAL FAT: 7G
CARBOHYDRATES: 45G
FIBER: 9G
PROTEIN: 10G

There's this American dream to put enough away that you can golf and build a birdhouse or just be in a Barcalounger watching football all day. I'll never be that guy. Our desires as men are to work, plow ahead, and overcome conflict. —KEVIN BACON

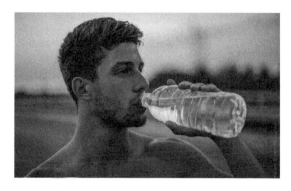

WATER

Water is absolutely crucial to nearly all your biological processes and makes up about 60 percent of your total body weight. Muscles themselves are 75 percent water. A general recommendation for water intake is 3 liters, or 12 cups per day, but not all water we consume comes from a glass. Fruit and vegetables offer our bodies water, too. On average we get about one liter (4 cups) from food, which leaves us with the classic recommendation of 8 cups per day. Obviously things like body size, climate, and activity level will affect the amount of water you need. Vigorous exercise can as much as double fluid requirements.

Thirst is a poor indicator of dehydration. Typically by the time you feel thirsty, you've already lost 1 to 2 percent of your body's water. Muscle strength will reduce with more significant water loss (closer to 4 percent).

Drink regularly, throughout the day, to stay hydrated and maintain the muscle mass you've worked so hard to build.

WORKOUT CLOTHES AND ACCESSORIES

When you dress for optimal fitness, it's essential to wear the right material and feel good about how you look. Here are a few of my basics.

SHIRTS

I prefer tank tops to shirts with any kind of sleeves because they give me a bit more freedom of movement and keep me a little cooler. Sweat is inevitable when you work out, so I opt for moisture-wicking fabrics, which carry sweat away from my body, minimizing chafing and general discomfort.

SHORTS

Compression shorts keep you in place while still allowing a full range of motion. Again, moisture-wicking fabrics provide maximum comfort.

SHOES

The most important quality in a shoe is comfort. I'm not a big fan of toe-drop shoes, where the heel is higher than the front of the shoe. These shoes force your pelvis into a forward tilt, which is not good for core stability or any movement. Unfortunately, this is the style of most shoes commercially available. I recommend looking for a neutral shoe or even going barefoot from time to time. If you have pronation or supination issues—i.e., if your ankles tend to roll inward or outward—go to a specialist who can help you figure out the best shoe for you. I like Nike Free and New Balance Minimus.

APPS

Calisthenics is an age-old fitness technique, but that doesn't mean you can't use modern technology to fine-tune it. A fitness tracker can help you keep track of your activity, nutrition, and other stats. I like the Fitbit Charge HR because it syncs with your heart rate so you can accurately monitor calories burned. I use it in conjunction with the nutrition app MyFitnessPal, which has a large database of foods and a simple interface, making it an easy and reliable way to track calories you take in versus calories you expend.

Dress with intent. Noted fitness—er, funny—expert Jerry Seinfeld joked that choosing sweatpants as casual wear tells the world, "I give up. I can't compete in normal society." You may have replaced your baggy cotton sweats with moisture-wicking polyblends, but the rules haven't changed: Save your sweat-managing gear for the activities that make you sweat.

For music, my favorite app is Spotify. You can create different playlists for different workouts or just search for whatever you feel like listening to at the moment.

HEADPHONES

Music can pump up a workout, but cords can tangle you up. The easy fix is a pair of wireless headphones. You get great tunes without worrying that you'll trip and fall while doing lunges or squats. My favorite wireless headphones are by Beats. They've got great sound and good battery life.

A BEATS PRIMER

AMP UP YOUR TRAINING WITH A GREAT PLAYLIST

Fitness is about improving the duration and quality of your life. It's the longest game there is, which means it's important to find ways to keep boredom at bay. One of the easiest methods is to change your tune—or, in this case, your *tunes*. The right playlist of songs can make all the difference to a workout.

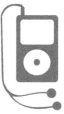 Lots of ready-made fitness compilations are built to deliver a steady rate of beats per minute. But that can get monotonous, especially if the songs aren't to your personal taste. The key to sustaining your interest and energy through a challenging workout isn't a uniform tempo—it's an absorbing narrative.

It may sound unconventional, but give it a try. Arrange your songs to tell a story, even if it's one that makes sense only to you. Choose music you feel a visceral response to, whether it's an urge to dance, an urge to cry, or just a powerful tug of nostalgia. Sequence the songs with the same care you put into making a mixtape (or Spotify playlist) for your first crush.

You'll want to see the story through to its conclusion even if your body is struggling, the same way you want to find out what happens at the end of a movie.

Start with a track with a long, portentous buildup, and end on an energetic anthem. Create playlists of different lengths for shorter and longer workouts. Include a dedicated track for warming up and one for cooling down. Transitions are key. You'll marvel at the power boost you feel when one great track flows seamlessly into another. Follow these tips or figure out whatever else works for you to keep you focused and present in the exercises. That's the best way to avoid injury and create the results you want.

TRACK 01 [WARMUP]
DAFFODILS
Mark Ronson
featuring Kevin Parker

TRACK 02
HARD TIMES (COVER)
John Legend and The Roots

TRACK 03
BRA
Cymande

TRACK 04
PASS THAT DUTCH
Missy Elliott

TRACK 05
MOVEMENT
LCD Soundsystem

TRACK 06
**LORD KNOWS /
FIGHTING STRONGER**
Meek Mill, Jhené Aiko
& Ludwig Goransson

TRACK 07
DANCING ON MY OWN
Robyn

TRACK 08 [COOLDOWN]
**GOD MOVING OVER
THE FACE OF THE WATERS**
Moby

THE WORKOUT PROGRAMS

AN OVERVIEW

Working out on your own can often be a challenge, not only in terms of staying motivated but also in terms of keeping your routines creative. The body adapts to exercise pretty easily. After eight weeks the body can make significant adaptations, and a given workout can become less effective. You want to keep your body guessing so that it has to work to continually adapt to whatever you throw at it. To do that, you need to keep changing up your strategy. The problem is that most people don't do this. They learn a few exercises and keep doing them over and over and over. Then they wonder why, if they're going to the gym four days a week, their gains have stalled. To combat routine ruts, I've developed three workout programs you can use in progression—or interchangeably if you're a seasoned exerciser—with lots of customization options to keep things fresh.

PROGRAM ONE
CONDITIONING

This four-week program, designed to condition, is aimed at someone who is relatively new to regular exercise. Each day provides a fully balanced workout that includes all the movement categories discussed earlier in the book. Begin with this program if you want to start with a balanced, full-body workout that also incorporates a good number of rest days to ensure proper recovery. If you're already in great shape and want to dive into more-advanced exercises from the get-go, you can skip this program and go straight to the second one.

PROGRAM TWO
STRENGTH BUILDING

This eight-week program, designed to build strength, involves a larger workload for the movement categories targeted, but with fewer categories per workout. It also has fewer rest days and a slower repetition tempo than Program One.

PROGRAM THREE
TOTAL BODY SHRED

This 12-week program, designed to help you achieve total-body fitness, alternates between conditioning workouts that focus on time rather than repetition and strength workouts with high intensity intervals built in. It's the culmination of the previous two programs and is a sustainable advanced workout.

CUSTOMIZING YOUR WORKOUT

One of the great things about calisthenics is that it's variable. I want you to be able to pick the workout program that works for you on any given day, depending on your location or access to certain pieces of equipment. In Program One, the four workouts are interchangeable, since they are all full-body balanced. If you find one of the workouts too difficult, replace it with another one from that program. Each workout in Program Two and Program Three offers a mix of push and pull movements that work the body vertically and/or horizontally, with some focusing on ankle-driven and others on hip-driven movements. These have been carefully planned to ensure balanced workouts over the course of weeks and months. If you want to swap an individual exercise for another one, just make sure they are from the same movement category.

KEEP IT INTERESTING

Varying your exercises is important to keep your body guessing and changing for the better, but another big hurdle we all have is a mental one. Your brain gets bored doing the same thing over and over in the same place. That's the beauty of bodyweight workouts. If you normally work out at home, go to the playground one day. When you're traveling, go to a park or the beach, or even use your hotel room. Work out with a friend; it's great to have someone else there pushing and motivating you. I also keep things fresh just by switching between different workout playlists.

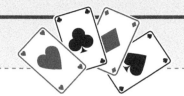

THE GAMBLER

> To keep realizing substantial benefits from your exercise, you'll need to vary your routine frequently. That isn't easy, but if the workout programs feel too structured for you, you can still get a balanced, if less formal, workout by using a deck of cards to prevent you from falling into a rut.

Choose four exercises, preferably one pushing move, one pulling move, one core exercise, and one ankle-driven exercise. Each exercise corresponds to one suit in the cards. Shuffle the deck, then turn over one card at a time. The suit and number of the card indicates what exercise and number of reps you perform. Face cards can indicate 5 reps (or 10 or 20 or whatever challenges you). Jokers should be something particularly arduous, like 20 burpees, or a sprint around the block. You can also sub in increments of time for reps; for example, each number on the card might indicate 10 seconds of planking time.

Try to complete the entire deck of cards as quickly as you can, with as little rest between sets as possible.

For example, you might choose for diamonds to represent pull-ups, hearts to represent push-ups, clubs to equal squats, and spades to equal crunches. A seven of diamonds means seven pull-ups. A four of hearts means four push-ups. Change at least two of the four exercises before your next Gambler's Workout—and, of course, shuffle the deck.

**TURN TO CHAPTER 8
for SPECIFICS ON ALL THREE
WORKOUT PROGRAMS**

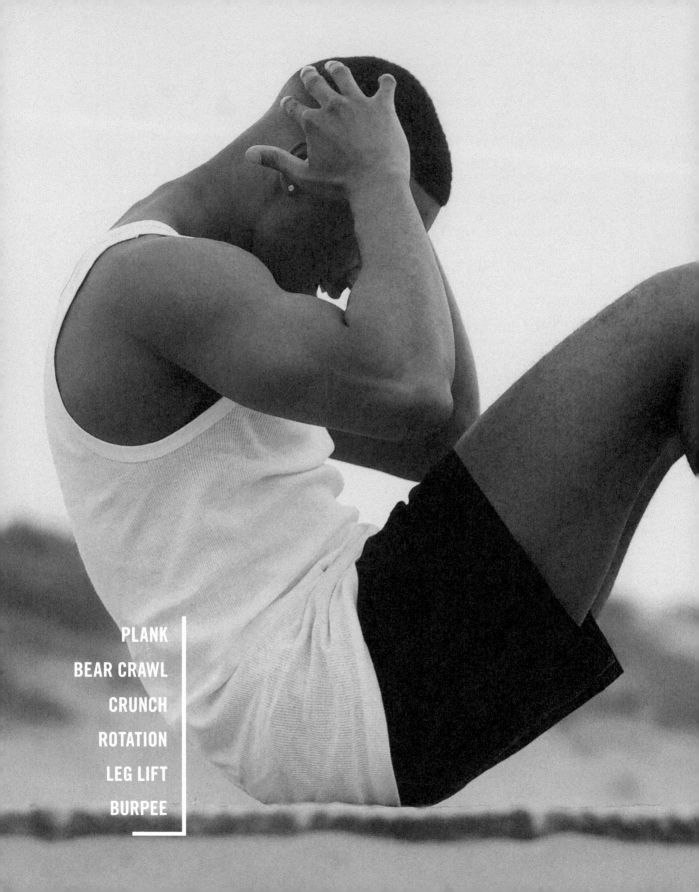

PLANK

BEAR CRAWL

CRUNCH

ROTATION

LEG LIFT

BURPEE

THREE

Think of your core as all the muscles between your knees and your chest—not just your abs. That includes the muscles around your pelvis, along your spine, and down your sides, as well as internal muscles you can't see in the mirror. Although your quadriceps aren't technically part of your core, many core exercises focus on the quadriceps, too, because they play a big role in

CORE

supporting core strength. Core musculature is important in many ways. It not only protects your vital organs but also provides an incredible amount of support and stability for all sorts of movement, from walking to leaning over to sitting up straight. When you lift heavy objects, it may seem like your arms are doing all the work, but your core is doing a lot, too. Trying to lift something heavy with a weak core is like trying to push a broken-down car while wearing roller skates: You can't generate the leverage you need. If you work on all your core muscles, instead of just your abs, you'll be stronger overall and less prone to injury. These exercises will help you do just that.

PLANK

Primary muscle groups: Abdominals, Obliques
Secondary muscle groups: Glutes, Quadriceps

—

01
BASE

CLASSIC PLANK

02
INTERMEDIATE

SIDE PLANK

03
ADVANCED

PLANK WALK-UP

The plank is an excellent exercise for making your spine more stable by fighting against gravity as it tries to pull your midsection down to the floor. There are many variations on the plank, but the goal is always the same: Use your abdominals to prevent your spine from arching, and use your glutes to prevent your pelvis from tilting forward. This plank series includes a classic plank to work the ab muscles that make up the six pack (rectus abdominis), a side plank to challenge the obliques, and finally, a plank walk-up to develop *reactive core stability*—the ability of your core to react to changes in demand or environment and continue to provide stability.

01 / CLASSIC PLANK

When your body is in a plank position, gravity tries to pull you to the floor. You feel its pull most strongly on the parts of your body that are farthest away from your feet and hands, which act as stable contact points with the ground. Because of this, your hips and lower back are the parts most vulnerable to gravity, and as they sag, your lower back increases its arch and your pelvis tilts forward. By engaging the abs and squeezing your glutes in a plank position, you can prevent the extension in your spine and the forward (anterior) tilt in your pelvis.

GOAL: Hold this position for at least 1 minute before moving to Plank Walk-Up (03).

1 Drop to the ground, and position yourself as if you were about to do a push-up: feet together, knees locked, and arms out straight in front of you. Your arms should be rotated outward with the insides of your elbows facing forward, and your shoulder blades should be pressed down toward your hips, not up around your ears. Your head should be neutral, not slumped down or extended back.

2 Squeeze your abdominals and glutes, and at the same time, tilt the top of your pelvis backward, rounding your lower back and taking any stress off of it by keeping your pelvis neutrally tilted. If you feel stress in your lower back, you don't have the right tilt to your pelvis yet. Your body should form a straight line from the top of your head through your shoulders, hips, knees, and ankles. (A) Hold this position for 30 seconds, gradually working up to be able to hold it for 1 minute.

Keep your knees locked and your neck neutral.

Drop your hips a little, one after the other, for an extra oblique burn.

Make sure your glutes and abs are clenching together.

Make sure your chest is long and your shoulder blades are pushed down.

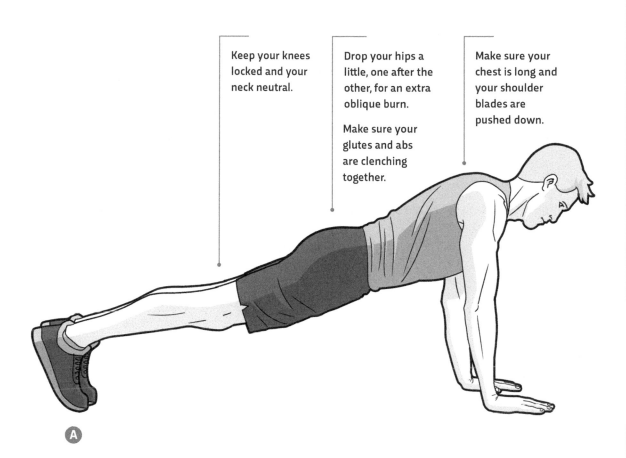

A

If your chest and shoulders are getting too tired, try doing the position with your elbows on the ground instead of your hands.

02 / SIDE PLANK

In this variation on the plank, you'll again use resistance to gravity to build strength in stability, but this time you'll be trying to keep your spine from bending sideways at the waist (lateral flexion). Engage your obliques and glutes to keep your pelvis and bottom leg in place.

GOAL: Hold this position for 1 minute on each side before moving to Plank Walk-Up (03).

1 Lie on your side with your legs straight and one foot on top of the other.

----

2 Using both arms, push yourself up until your bottom arm is stretched out straight, supporting all your upper body weight, and your top arm is lying on the upper side of your body. Make sure that both shoulder blades are pulled down toward your hips and that the supporting arm is rotated outward, with the inside of the elbow facing out in front of you.

----

3 Fully extend your hips by pushing them forward and squeezing your glutes. Your body should be a straight line from your ear through your shoulder, hips, knees, and ankles. **A**

----

4 Hold this position for 30 seconds, and repeat on the other side, gradually working up to be able to hold it for 1 minute on each side.

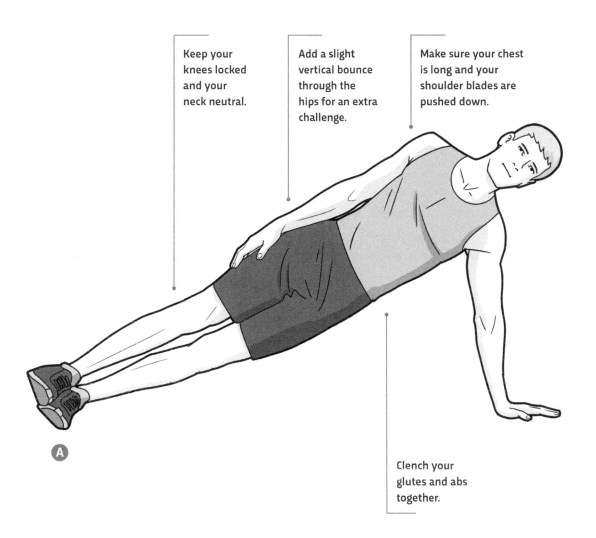

Keep your knees locked and your neck neutral.

Add a slight vertical bounce through the hips for an extra challenge.

Make sure your chest is long and your shoulder blades are pushed down.

A

Clench your glutes and abs together.

03 / PLANK WALK-UP

This plank variation challenges your reactive core stability and your ability to keep your spine and hips from twisting or rotating (antirotation). For a plank walk-up, you reduce your base of support by lifting one hand and placing it up on a step in front of you. This lack of support makes it easier for gravity to pull your spine into extension, and your core has to work extra hard to hold your spine in place. As you follow with the second hand, a whole new section of your trunk becomes more unstable and vulnerable to gravity.

GOAL: With practice, be able to perform at least 10 cycles on each side.

1 Start in a plank position with your hands 12 to 18 inches away from a sturdy step or curb. **A** (The higher the step, or the farther the distance, the more difficult the exercise.)

----

2 Lift your right hand, and place it on the step. **B** Then lift your left hand, and place it next to your right hand on the step, making sure not to rotate or tilt through the hips. **C**

----

3 Return your right hand to its original position, followed by your left hand. **D E**

----

4 Switch, and lead with the left hand. Repeat each side for five reps.

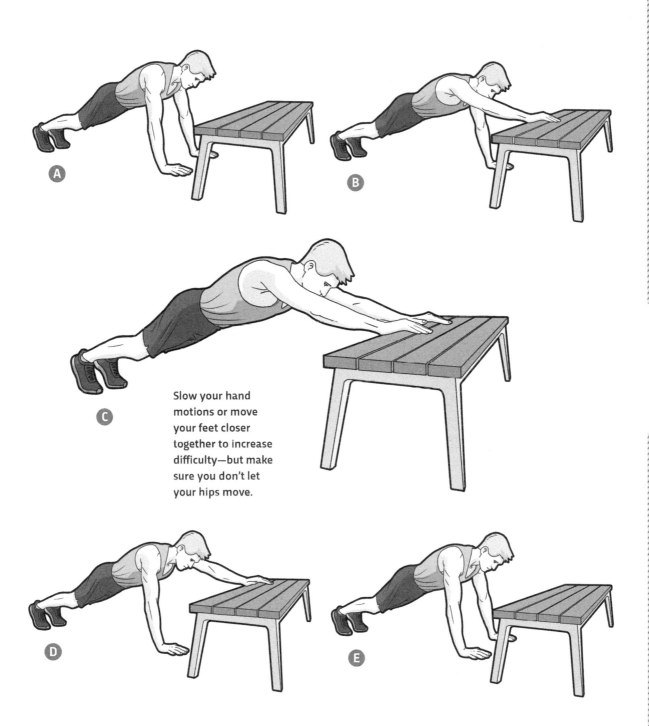

Slow your hand motions or move your feet closer together to increase difficulty—but make sure you don't let your hips move.

BEAR CRAWL

Primary muscle groups: Deltoids, Hip flexors, Abdominals
Secondary muscle groups: Obliques, Hamstrings

04

BASE

FORWARD BEAR CRAWL

05

INTERMEDIATE

LATERAL CRAB WALK

06

ADVANCED

GLANIMAL CRAWL

You probably mastered this fundamental movement pattern before you learned to walk, but you may have forgotten it by now. The bear crawl challenges your core to prevent unwanted movement as you use your limbs in contralateral (opposite-side) unison. Here you'll practice crawling forward with your spine neutral, then progress to a more difficult variation where you'll switch up your movement and crawl laterally from side to side. For the hardest variation, you'll return to a forward bear crawl with longer strides and some rotation allowed through the hips and shoulders.

04 / FORWARD BEAR CRAWL

The goal of a basic bear crawl is to crawl forward while preventing any motion in your spine. Your right arm always moves at the same time as your left leg, and vice versa. Your hips and knees drive your motion forward, while your arms absorb the impact with the ground, slowing your motion and providing extra stability. Your spine, pelvis, and head remain neutral.

GOAL: Strive to be able to complete 20 to 30 repetitions on each side.

1 Drop to the ground on all fours with your hands below your shoulders and your knees below your hips.

---

2 Position your pelvis so the lower region of your spine is in neutral, then lift your chest and activate your lower-trapezius muscles by pressing your shoulder blades down toward your hips.

---

3 Lift your knees 1 inch off the ground, and when you're ready, move your left arm and right leg forward together 4 to 5 inches. (A) Then do the same thing but with your right arm and left leg. (B) Repeat 10 times.

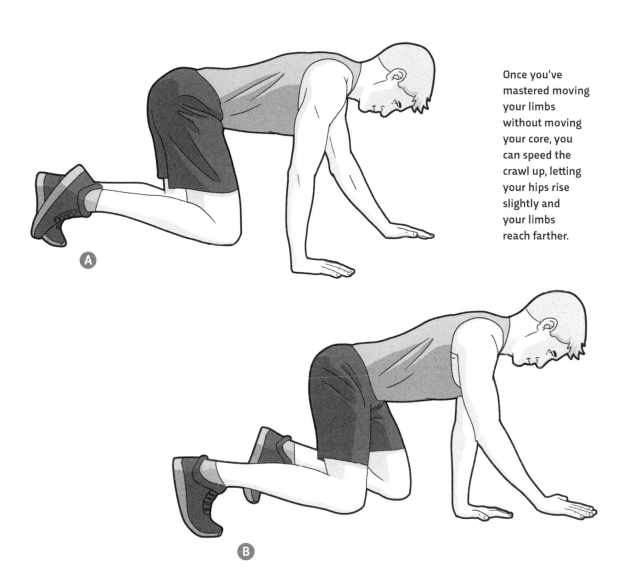

Once you've mastered moving your limbs without moving your core, you can speed the crawl up, letting your hips rise slightly and your limbs reach farther.

A

B

05 / LATERAL CRAB WALK

This variation of the bear crawl starts from a plank position (01) instead of on all fours. As in the forward bear crawl (04), you move your arms and legs opposite each other in unison, but this time, you make your way from side to side instead of forward. Engage your abdominals to prevent your spine and hips from sagging and to provide stability for your moving limbs.

GOAL: Work to be able to complete 10 to 15 repetitions in each direction.

1 Start in a plank position, with your hands shoulder-width apart and your feet together. Make sure there's enough space clear to your left for you to travel in that direction. A

2 Lift your right arm and left leg at the same time, bringing your hands together and moving your left leg to create a space roughly equal to shoulder width. B

3 Now with your hands together and your feet apart, move your left arm and your right leg at the same time to complete one repetition. C This movement will return you to the starting plank position, except now you're a couple feet to the left. Repeat five times, then perform the movement in the opposite direction for five reps.

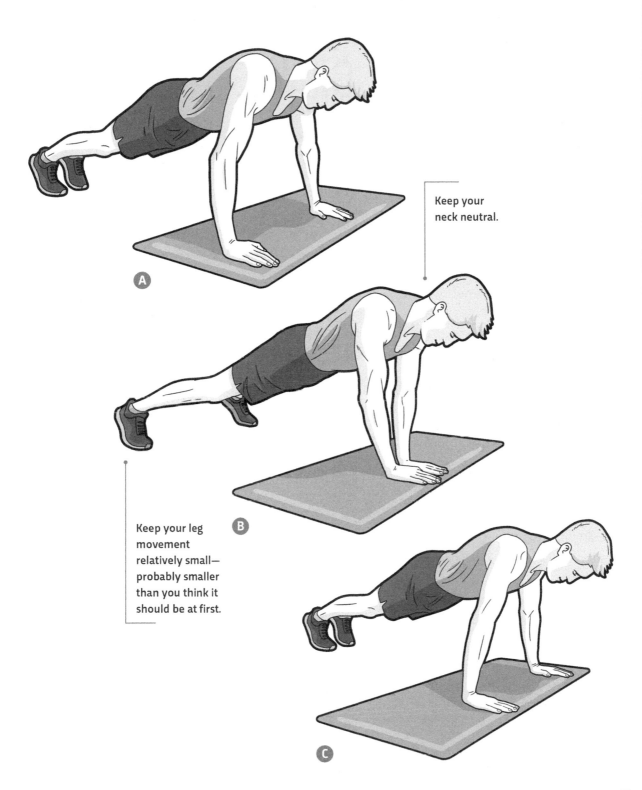

Keep your
neck neutral.

Keep your leg
movement
relatively small—
probably smaller
than you think it
should be at first.

A

B

C

06 / GLANIMAL CRAWL

In this harder version of the bear crawl—named after my friend Glen, who is a total animal—you still move your arms and legs opposite each other in unison, but with much more exaggerated motions, dropping your body down almost to the ground. When you drive your weight off your hands to initiate the motion forward and backward, you work the pushing muscles in your upper body. The real challenge is the reverse portion of the set, when you try to retrace your steps without having to reposition any of your limbs.

GOAL: Try for 20 to 30 repetitions on each side.

1 Drop to the ground on all fours with your hands below your shoulders and your knees below your hips. **A**

----

2 Bring your right foot closer to your right hand, and extend your left arm and left leg as far as they can go, dropping your torso to within a few inches of the ground. **B**

----

3 Lift your right arm and left leg together, and press off the right leg and left arm, **C** covering as much ground as you can.

----

4 Start with five repetitions on each side, then retrace your steps backward, trying not to make extra contact with the ground.

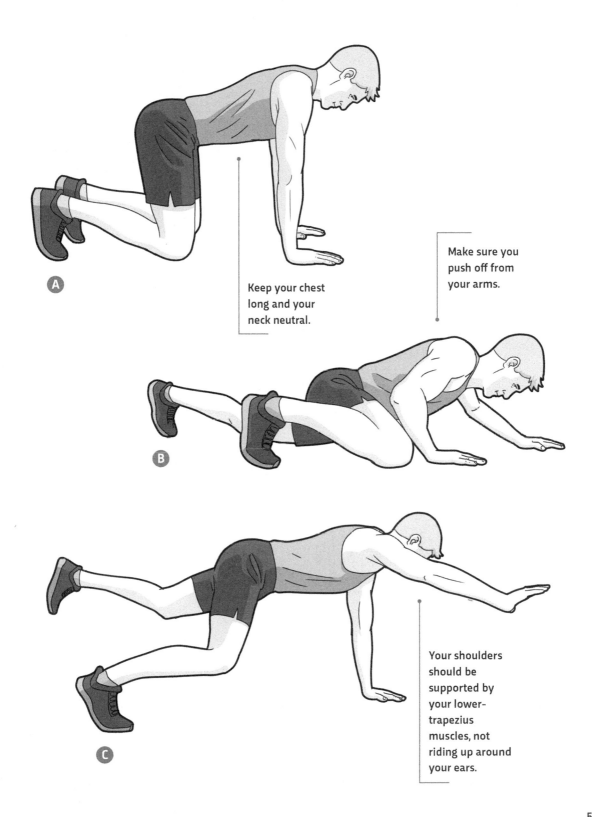

A

Keep your chest long and your neck neutral.

Make sure you push off from your arms.

B

C

Your shoulders should be supported by your lower-trapezius muscles, not riding up around your ears.

CRUNCH

Primary muscle groups: Abdominals, Hip flexors
Secondary muscle group: Obliques

07

BASE

CLASSIC CRUNCH

08

INTERMEDIATE

OBLIQUE CRUNCH

09

ADVANCED

V-UP

Typically you use your core to prevent motion, not create it. But besides helping you drop body fat, crunches can be one of the best ways to create muscle definition and build a six- or eight-pack. There are many schools of thought these days that say you can achieve a six-pack without crunches and that crunches may actually do more harm than good, because if your form isn't perfect, they can put a lot of strain on your spine. Defined abs aren't worth a herniated disc. I tend to agree with these criticisms to some extent, but I still see a point in including them in this book. I won't be including any crunches in the workout programs (chapter 8), but if you understand the risks and have a low enough body-fat percentage to see definition in your abs, feel free to substitute crunches for any of my core exercises.

07 / CLASSIC CRUNCH

The classic crunch can be done in many ways. For our purposes, you'll do it with your knees bent and your feet on the ground, targeting your abs as you raise your chest up toward the ceiling. Remember that it's just as important to control the elongation of your abs as you return to the starting position as it is when crunching upward, so make sure you're in control throughout the entire motion.

GOAL: 20 repetitions with perfect form

1 Start on your back with your knees bent and your feet flat on the ground. Place your hands behind your ears (so you're not tempted to pull on the back of your head). **A**

----

2 Sit up, trying to bring your chest toward the ceiling rather than toward your knees. **B** Exhale sharply to fully evacuate your lungs.

----

3 Once you've come up as high as you can, slowly inhale and return to your starting position in a controlled manner until your head is back on the ground.

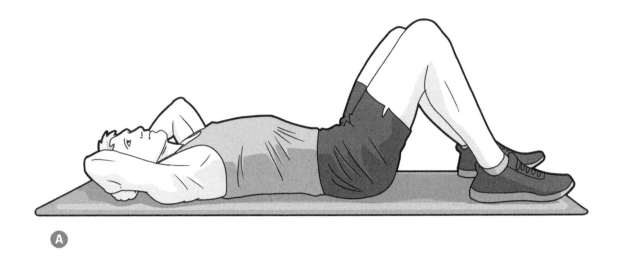

A

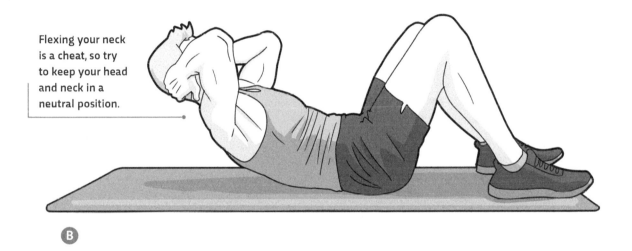

Flexing your neck is a cheat, so try to keep your head and neck in a neutral position.

B

08 / OBLIQUE CRUNCH

This crunch variation targets the oblique muscles located on the outside of the abdominals. The obliques are those diagonal, finger-shaped muscles that complement the six-pack so well, and they help you rotate your torso, too. This exercise targets one side at a time, so don't alternate with each rep. Continue working one side until it's exhausted.

GOAL: 20 repetitions on each side

1 Start by lying on your back with your knees bent and your feet flat on the ground. Turn your lower body to the right so the bottom knee is on the floor, while keeping both shoulders on the ground. Place your hands behind your ears (so you're not tempted pull on the back of your head). **A**

2 Crunch upward toward the ceiling, exhaling sharply to fully evacuate your lungs. **B** Slowly inhale, and return to your starting position in a controlled manner.

3 Start by repeating on the same side 10 times, then switching to the other side.

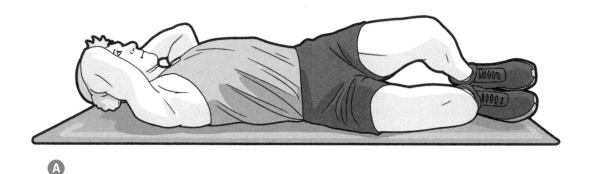

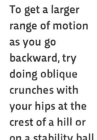

To get a larger range of motion as you go backward, try doing oblique crunches with your hips at the crest of a hill or on a stability ball.

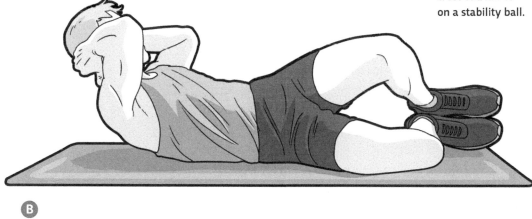

09 / V-UP

The V-up is a cross between a leg raise and a crunch, and it's a huge challenge for your abdominal muscles. Because of the modified V-shape you use as your starting position, your abs have to fight for stability as you lower your limbs toward the ground and then bring them back up. It also requires you to bring your arms overhead, which is a great way to maintain shoulder mobility.

GOAL: Aim to get your legs within a few inches of the ground and/or do 20 repetitions.

1 Start by lying on your back with your arms and legs pointed up toward the ceiling so that your body is roughly in the shape of a V. **A**

2 Keeping your legs straight, slowly lower them toward the ground while at the same time lowering your arms toward the ground over your head. **B** Keep your abs tight so that your lower back never arches up off the ground.

3 When your abs can no longer hold your back to the ground and it starts to arch upward, stop the descent and crunch your arms and legs back up to the starting position, keeping them straight the whole time.

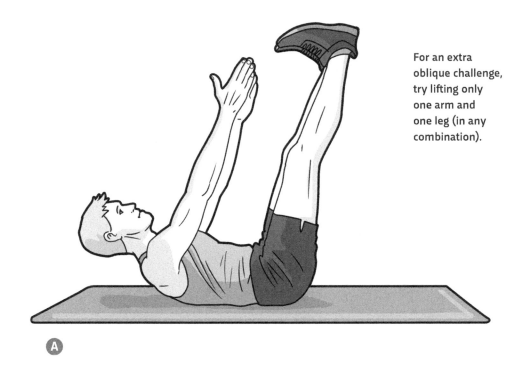

For an extra oblique challenge, try lifting only one arm and one leg (in any combination).

A

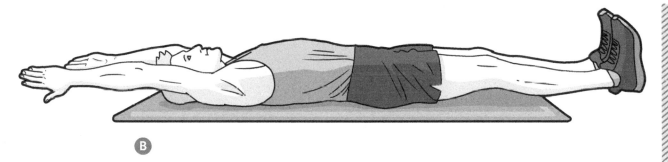

B

ROTATION

Primary muscle groups: Abdominals, Obliques
Secondary muscle group: Hip flexors

10
BASE
BICYCLE

11
INTERMEDIATE
WINDSHIELD WIPER

12
ADVANCED
PLANK WITH ROTATIONAL KICK-THROUGH

One major function of the core muscles is to keep you stable and strong both when your torso is turning (rotational) and when it resists turning and stays still (antirotational). For these exercises, you want to be rotating from the middle, or thoracic, region of the spine—the section where your ribs attach—not the lower, or lumbar, region. Strive to keep your lower spine and pelvis neutral. These exercises will build your controlled rotational stability with progressively harder movements, finishing with a plank-based exercise for an extra stability challenge.

10 / BICYCLE

Bicycles challenge your obliques by rotating one shoulder toward the opposite hip. You guide the motion by reaching your elbow toward the opposite knee, keeping your hands positioned behind your head. Bicycles do work your abs, but don't think of them as crunches. Instead, focus on the rotation of your spine.

GOAL: Work up to 20 repetitions on each side before attempting the Windshield Wiper (11).

1 Lie flat on your back with your hands behind your ears and your knees bent. Lift your feet, keeping your abs tight, so that your hips form a 90-degree angle and your knees form a 45-degree angle.

2 Extend your right leg out as if straightening it. (You don't have to get it perfectly straight.) At the same time, rotate through your core to bring your right elbow toward your left knee. **A**

3 Slowly retract your right leg while simultaneously extending your left leg and bringing your left elbow toward your right knee as it arrives back at its starting position. **B**

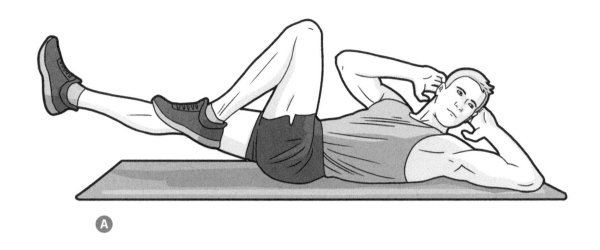

A

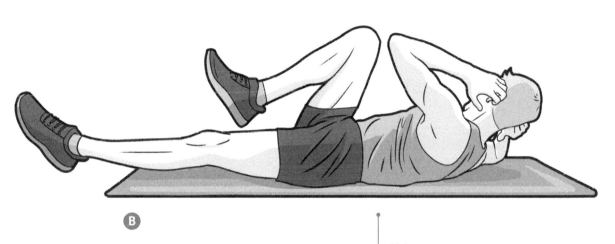

B

Make sure not
to round your
lower spine.

11 / WINDSHIELD WIPER

In this exercise, you'll develop your obliques by lying on your back and moving your legs from side to side like windshield wipers. Try not to push off the ground with your arms—instead, rely only on your core's strength and control. Make sure you're getting all your rotation from the middle of your spine. Your spine's lower region should maintain its natural curve, even if that means you have to keep your knees bent. Straighten your legs only if you can maintain your lower spine's curve through the entire motion.

GOAL: Try for 20 repetitions on each side.

1 Lie flat on your back with your legs straight up in the air. Put your arms out to your sides with your palms up. **A**

2 Keeping your feet together, slowly lower your legs to the right, as if your legs were slow, controlled windshield wipers. **B** Stop when your opposite shoulder starts to rise up off the ground.

3 In a controlled motion, reverse direction and bring your legs back to the starting position. **A** Repeat on the left. **C**

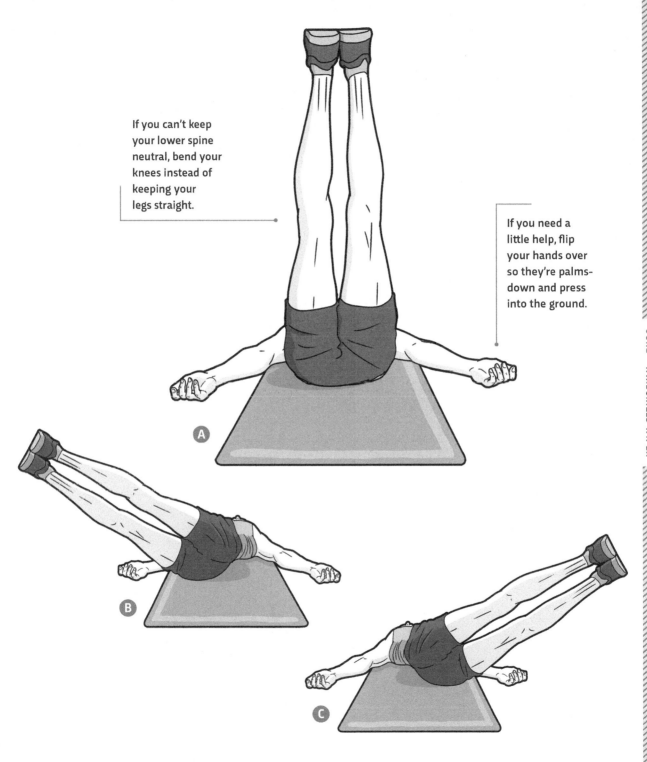

If you can't keep your lower spine neutral, bend your knees instead of keeping your legs straight.

If you need a little help, flip your hands over so they're palms-down and press into the ground.

A

B

C

12 / PLANK WITH ROTATIONAL KICK-THROUGH

This move combines a rotational exercise with the stability challenge of a plank (01) to work your entire core. You start in a plank position, then slowly kick one leg under the other and out the other side. The kick doesn't have to be particularly high, but the higher you get it, the more of a squeeze you'll feel in your obliques. Make sure your glutes and abs are firing to keep any pressure from reaching the lower back, and let your shoulders and shoulder blades move a little to ensure you're rotating through the middle of your spine.

GOAL: 20 repetitions on each side

1 Start in a plank position. **A** Drop your left hip and shoulder as you start to kick your left leg under your right leg and straight out the other side.

---

2 As you rotate, drop the inside edge of your right leg and kick through with your left heel, locking your left knee. **B**

---

3 Slowly rotate back to the plank position, bringing your left leg back from under your right leg to its original position. **A** Repeat on the right side. **C**

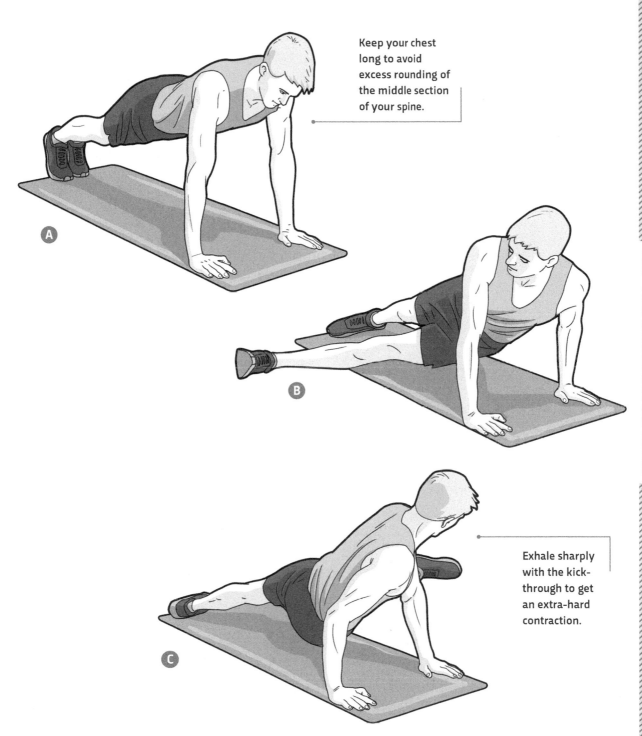

Keep your chest long to avoid excess rounding of the middle section of your spine.

A

B

Exhale sharply with the kick-through to get an extra-hard contraction.

C

CORE   PLANK WITH ROTATIONAL KICK-THROUGH

67

LEG LIFT

Primary muscle groups: Abdominals, Hip flexors
Secondary muscle group: Obliques

13

BASE

SUPINE
LEG RAISE

14

INTERMEDIATE

HANGING
LEG RAISE

15

INTERMEDIATE

PLANK
WITH
ROTATIONAL
KNEE TUCK

Raising and lowering your legs is a great way to challenge the stability of your abs and your lower spine. As you raise or lower your legs, either when you start on the ground or from a hanging position, you can feel the lower portion of your spine start to arch into extension as your legs pull your pelvis into a forward tilt. It's your abdominals' job to prevent that extension and tilt from happening. Here you'll start by doing leg lifts while lying on the floor, progress to doing them while hanging from a bar, and eventually work up to doing them from a plank position. All three variations require tons of abdominal activation to keep the lower spine stable, so no matter which exercise you're on, you'll be building muscle and improving your core strength.

13 / SUPINE LEG RAISE

Supine simply means "lying flat on your back." In this particular exercise, you'll start by lying down with your legs straight up in the air, then lowering them as comfortably as you can until they're parallel to the ground. Make sure your abdominals do their job and keep your lower spine neutral against the floor. Try not to press your arms into the floor for added stability—this move is for your abs, not your arms. If you feel your back coming up off the floor, stop your legs where they are. You don't need to get your legs perfectly horizontal on your first try. Just work the range of motion under your control until you have the strength to take it further.

GOAL: Increase your range of motion until you can lower your feet to a point just above the floor. You want to be able to do 20 repetitions before you try the Hanging Leg Raise (14).

1 Lie flat on your back with your legs pointed straight up in the air. **A** Inhale as you slowly lower your legs **B** until your lower spine starts to rise up off the floor.

- -

2 Exhale as you raise your legs back up to the starting position. Repeat 10 times.

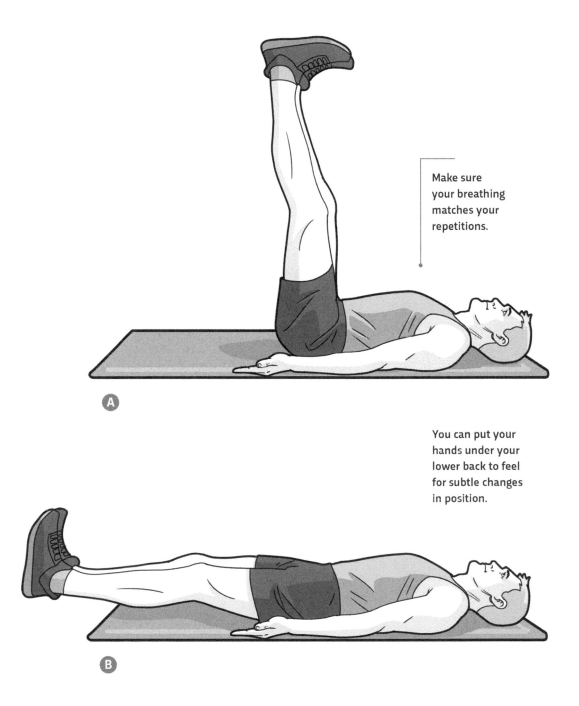

Make sure your breathing matches your repetitions.

A

You can put your hands under your lower back to feel for subtle changes in position.

B

14 / HANGING LEG RAISE

The hanging leg raise works best when the bar you're hanging from is high enough that you can fully extend your arms and legs. For this exercise, you'll try to raise your legs to horizontal (or higher) and then return them to their starting position without letting your body swing backward. You can use an open, closed, or mixed grip, whichever is more comfortable for you. Just make sure you grip hard enough with your hands to activate your shoulders, and keep your shoulders pulled down toward your hips to protect your shoulder joints.

GOAL: As you get stronger, try to raise your legs past horizontal—all the way to the height of the bar, if you can.

1 Hang from the bar while lowering your shoulder blades toward your hips to engage your lower-trapezius muscles. **A**

2 Exhale as you raise your legs as high as you can in front of you with your knees locked. **B**

3 Inhale as you lower your legs in a controlled manner to prevent swinging. Engage your abdominals to prevent extension in your lower spine.

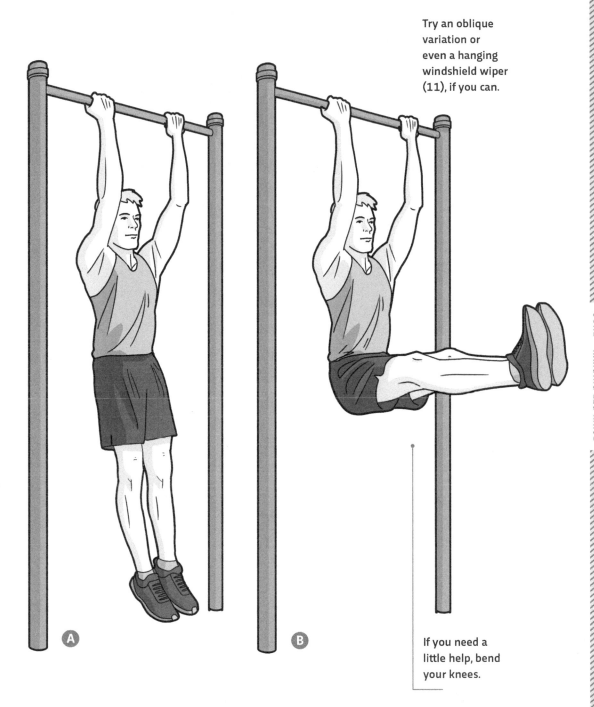

Try an oblique variation or even a hanging windshield wiper (11), if you can.

If you need a little help, bend your knees.

A

B

15 / PLANK WITH ROTATIONAL KNEE TUCK

To give you an extra stability challenge, this version of the leg raise is done in a plank position (01) on a smooth floor with a towel under your feet. If you don't have a towel on hand, you can use a paper towel, a paper plate, or anything else that will slide along the floor. From the plank position, you drop one hip slightly and tuck both your knees up toward your chest. Try to exhale completely as you finish the tuck and inhale as you return to the plank position.

GOAL: **20 repetitions on each side**

1 Start in a plank position on a hard, smooth surface with a towel under your feet. **A**

---

2 Slightly drop your left hip, and pull both your knees up toward your chest on the right side. **B** The towel lets your feet slide so you can keep the movement smooth and controlled.

---

3 Keeping your abs engaged, level out your hips and straighten your legs back into a plank position. **A** Repeat on the left side. **C**

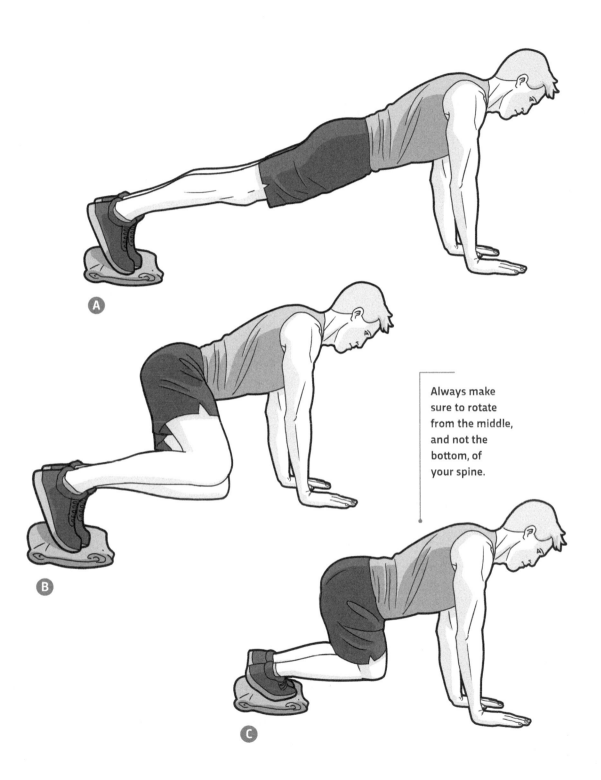

Always make
sure to rotate
from the middle,
and not the
bottom, of
your spine.

BURPEE

Primary muscle groups: Abdominals, Pectorals, Deltoids, Quadriceps, Glutes, Hamstrings

16
BASE

ELEVATED BURPEE

17
INTERMEDIATE

CLASSIC BURPEE

18
ADVANCED

ONE ARM BURPEE

The burpee in all its forms is one of the best full-body bodyweight exercises out there. With its wide range of movements—hip-hinging, squatting, planking, and pushing—it works almost all the muscle groups in your body, but it's particularly great for your core. With so many motions, there's a lot that can go wrong, so it's important to learn the correct form. Here you'll start with a slightly easier version so you can master the right movements. Then you'll move on to the classic burpee, and then to something a little more difficult if you want to really challenge yourself.

16 / ELEVATED BURPEE

A slightly easier version of the classic burpee, the elevated burpee is performed in front of a step, so you don't need as much ankle and hip mobility for the squat (19) or as much core strength to stabilize you during the plank phase (01). Instead of bringing your hands all the way to the ground while hinging and squatting, you're just bringing them down far enough to reach the elevated step. This lets your lower (lumbar) spine remain more neutral, rather than forcing it into flexion repeatedly. The higher the step, the easier the burpee, so make sure you're challenging yourself appropriately.

GOAL: **Maintain a neutral lower spine through the entire range of movement. Once you can do 20 repetitions, move on to the Classic Burpee (17).**

1 Start by standing about 12 inches in front of your chosen step with your feet hip-width apart. A

2 While maintaining a neutral spine, drop into a squat, put your arms straight out in front of you, and place your hands on top of the step. B

3 Once your hands are securely on the step, hop your feet out behind you, landing in a plank position. C

4 Hop your legs forward, returning to the spot in front of the step that you started with, landing in a squat position. B

5 Keeping your chest tall and your back straight, press through your legs and return to a standing position. A

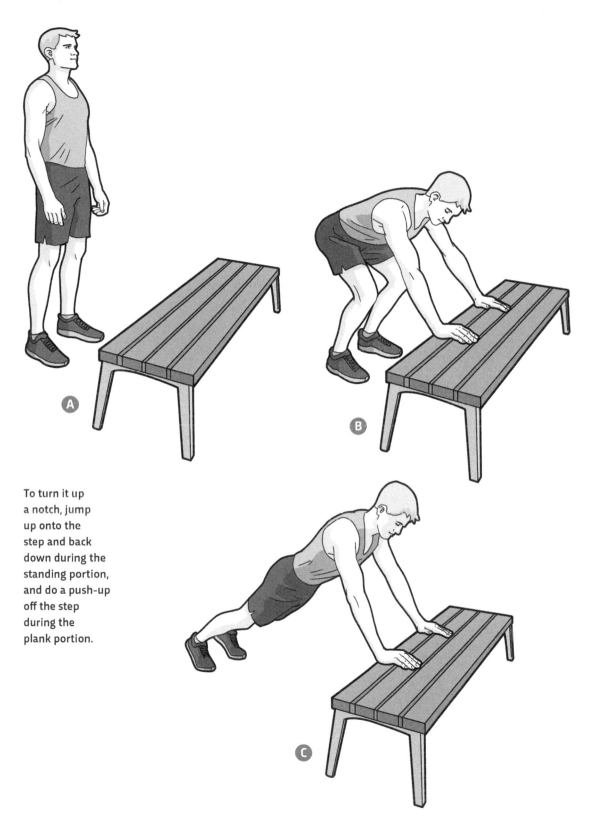

To turn it up a notch, jump up onto the step and back down during the standing portion, and do a push-up off the step during the plank portion.

17 / CLASSIC BURPEE

This burpee is done without the assistance of an elevated surface, so you have to hinge and squat (19) all the way to the ground. Remember that on the way down and the way up, your knees must stay out over your feet and not collapse inward. This collapse is a dangerous compensation and can lead to serious injury. If this is something you do without thinking, you should train yourself out of the habit immediately. Your hips and ankles need to be properly stabilized to perform any ankle-driven or explosive movements, and the burpee involves both. For proper squat form, see illustration B on page 93.

GOAL: 20 repetitions

1 Squat with your feet hip-width apart. Bend forward with your arms straight below you, keeping your back straight until your hands reach the ground. **A**

2 Once your hands are secured, hop your feet out behind you, landing in a plank position. **B**

3 Hop forward from the plank position, returning to a deep squat position, **A** and lift your hands so they're no longer on the floor.

4 Keeping your chest tall and your back straight, press through your legs to a standing position with your arms raised above your head. **C**

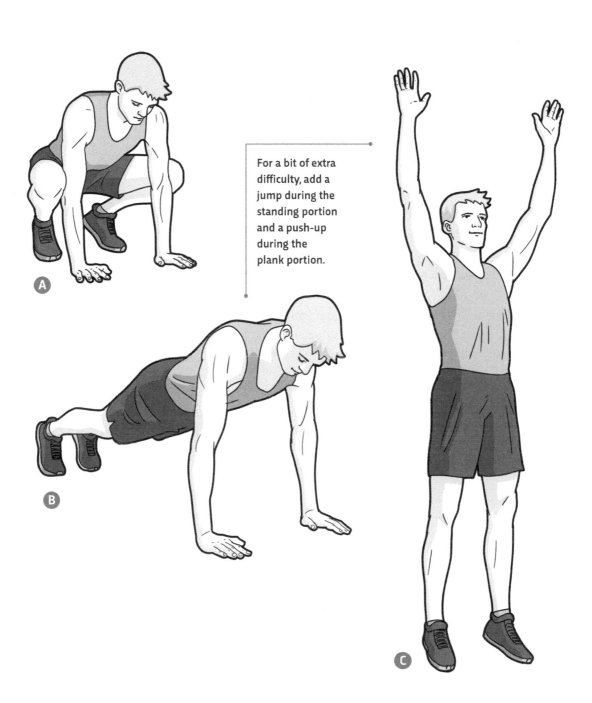

For a bit of extra difficulty, add a jump during the standing portion and a push-up during the plank portion.

A

B

C

18 / ONE ARM BURPEE

The one arm burpee is exactly what it sounds like. It involves the same motions as a classic burpee (17), but instead of using both arms during the plank portion (01), you use only one. Because you're decreasing your support base from two hands to one, your core has to work harder to keep you stable. (The one arm you're using has to work harder as well since it has no help from the other arm.) You can start with the elevated variation or go straight to the ground. Just make sure you follow all the requirements for a burpee: Keep your knees over your feet, and keep your lower spine as neutral as possible.

GOAL: 10 repetitions on each arm

1 Stand with your feet hip-width apart. Squat and bend forward with your left arm straight below you, keeping your back straight until your left hand reaches the ground. **A**

2 Once your hand is secure, hop your feet out behind you, landing in a one-handed plank position. **B**

3 Hop forward from the plank position, returning to a deep squat position, **C** and lift your hand so it's no longer on the floor.

4 Keeping your chest long and your back straight, press through your legs and return to a standing position. **D** Repeat using your right hand.

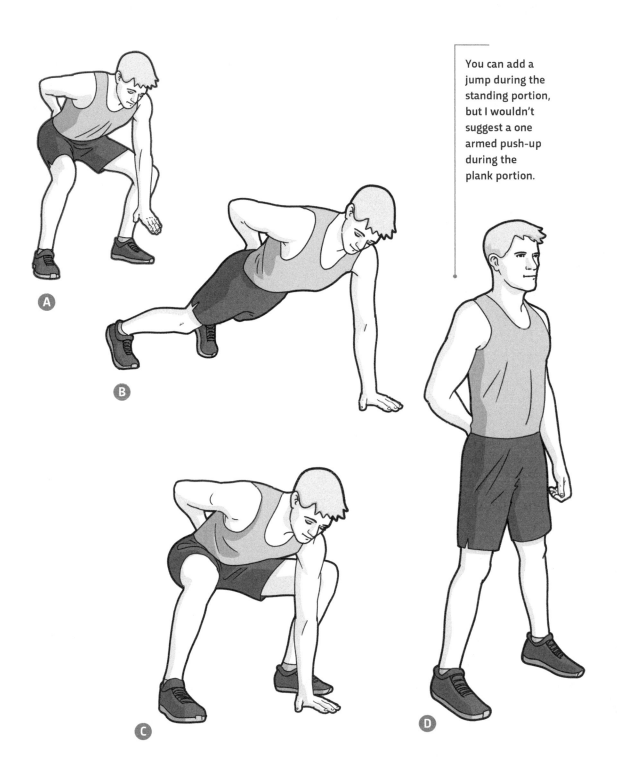

You can add a jump during the standing portion, but I wouldn't suggest a one armed push-up during the plank portion.

A

B

C

D

SQUAT

LUNGE

STEP-UP

JUMP

DYNAMIC JUMP

FOUR

In ankle-driven movements, you bend at the ankle, moving your shin forward over the top of your foot. This movement—called dorsiflexion—forces your hips and ankles to provide more stabilization and increases the demands on your calves, quads, and glutes. It also gives your knee a much larger range of motion than it has during, say, hip-driven exercises. Form may vary, and

ANKLE DRIVEN

some lunge patterns may not have as much bend at the ankle, but I still consider them ankle-driven and always encourage my clients to practice at least some healthy forward movement of the shin and knee during their lunges. It helps create good movement habits and elasticity through the lower leg, which strengthens your ankles and tones your leg muscles.

SQUAT

Primary muscle groups: Quadriceps, Hamstrings, Glutes
Secondary muscle groups: Calves, Abdominals, Spinal erectors

19

BASE

SQUAT

20

INTERMEDIATE

SPLIT
SQUAT

21

ADVANCED

REAR
ELEVATED
SPLIT SQUAT

One of the most functional movements of any workout routine, the squat is the best way to get to the ground and up. The squat burns tons of calories and, when done correctly, challenges both your upper body's stability and your legs' mobility, so you get a core workout while you work on your quads and glutes. A correct squat distributes your weight evenly between the heels and the balls of your feet and positions your spine parallel with your shin bone (tibia). Once you've mastered the basic move, you can push yourself even harder with variations like the one-sided split squat and the high-intensity rear elevated split squat.

19 / SQUAT

Most of us know what a squat looks like, but it's not quite as simple as it seems. If you want to avoid injury and really sculpt your thighs and glutes, there are a few things to pay attention to. Feet don't need to be parallel but should ideally be no more than 15 degrees out. However, the shin bone and knees *do* need to come straight over the midline of the foot, matching whichever angle you've decided to use. The arch of your foot should not collapse. If your toes are forced wider as you descend, you most likely need to work on your ankle mobility (calf stretches can help). Your knees can come out over your toes as long as you have enough ankle mobility and your weight stays evenly distributed between the balls of your feet and your heels. If you need to put your arms out in front to balance, that's okay, but strive for the mobility to keep your weight centered without using your arms as a counterbalance.

GOAL: You want to get your shin bone parallel with your spine at the bottom of the squat. Do 20 repetitions. Form is everything on this exercise.

1 Stand with your feet shoulder-width apart (or slightly wider if needed) and within 15 degrees of parallel. **A**

----

2 While keeping a tall chest, bend your knees and begin to squat as low as you can while still maintaining control of the movement, or until the tops of your thighs are parallel with the ground. **B** Make sure to keep your weight evenly distributed between your heels and the balls of your feet.

----

3 Press through your heel and midfoot and rise, with your hips and shoulders moving as one unit, back to your starting position. **A**

Make your squat easier or harder by varying your arm positions. Try doing squats with your arms by your sides, out in front, or up over your head.

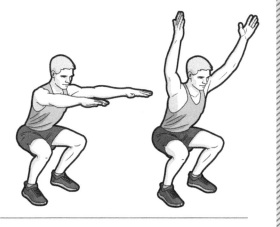

Keep your spine stable and resist bending.

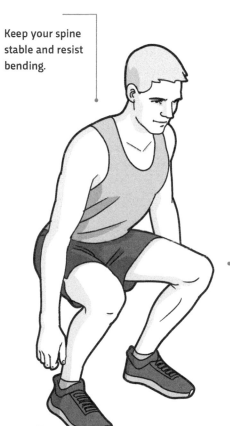

Do wall sits to help build stability: With your back to a wall, feet shoulder-width apart, squat down, keeping your back against the wall until your knees are bent to 90 degrees and positioned directly above your feet.

If you have trouble keeping your arches tall and your feet stationary, keep your squat shallow until you have enough mobility to go deeper.

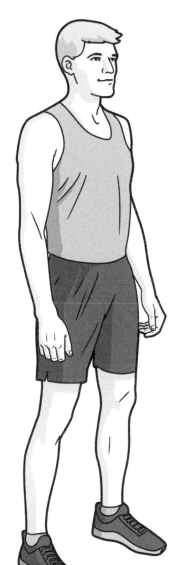

A

B

20 / SPLIT SQUAT

A split squat keeps both feet stationary like a regular squat, but it starts from a staggered foot position, where one is out in front of the other. The ideal distance between your feet is whatever distance brings your back hip to a neutral position at the bottom of the squat. To figure out how far that is for you, start your split squats from a comfortable half-kneeling position until you're more familiar with the movement. This is a good way to practice hip stability before moving on to lunges.

GOAL: Try to keep your feet parallel and your spine vertical throughout all your repetitions. Once you can do 20 repetitions on each side with perfect form, try out the Rear Elevated Split Squat (21).

1 Get down on one knee and start in a half-kneel with your bottom knee lined up under your hip and your hip lined up under your shoulder. Plant your front foot firmly on the ground, relatively close to the bottom knee. **A**

2 Keeping your spine vertical, press through both feet and rise to a split stance with both feet flat on the ground, one out in front of the other. **B**

3 Try to maintain your balance as you slowly return to the half-kneel position. **A**

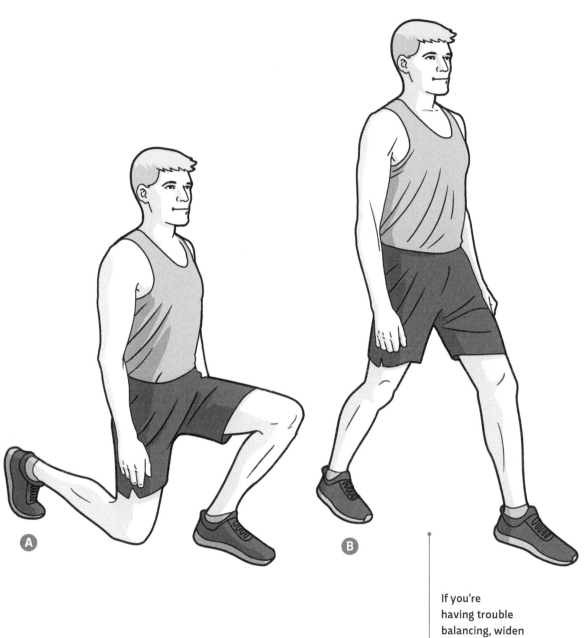

A

B

If you're having trouble balancing, widen your foot base.

21 / REAR ELEVATED SPLIT SQUAT

In this variation of the split squat, the rear leg is raised up behind you on a chair, bench, or other object so it can't contribute to the raising and lowering of your body. Make sure you have something to grab onto when you first try this one, as it can be a challenge to keep your balance throughout the entire motion—but that challenge is what gives you strong thighs, glutes, and core muscles. It's very important to make sure the hip on the working leg stays in line with your shoulder, knee, and ankle. Otherwise, you may just be reinforcing bad movement mechanics and opening yourself up to injuries.

GOAL: 20 repetitions on each side

1 Elevate one foot behind you on a step or bench, preferably with your foot flat and your toes pointed back, so that the tops of your toes rest on the step or bench. **A**

2 Hop out on the standing leg until you start to feel a stretch in the hip flexor of the back leg. That means you're in the right position.

3 Slowly lower yourself on the standing leg until the top of your thigh is parallel with the ground. **B**

4 Drive up through the standing leg only and return to your starting position. **A**

If you're having trouble with balance, do this squat variation near a wall or another object you can use to steady yourself.

Try to keep your body upright, and don't let your hips sway out to the side.

Try to keep your pelvis neutral and your lower back stable throughout the entire motion.

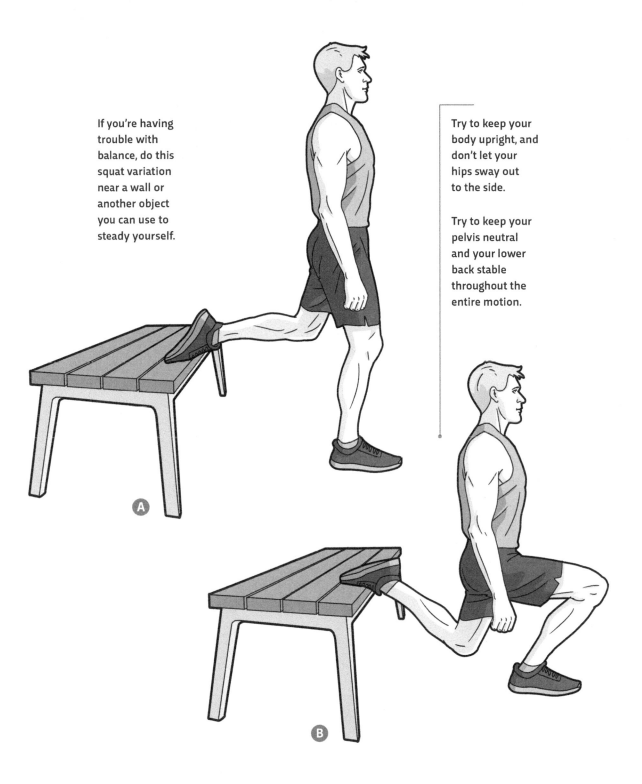

A

B

LUNGE

Primary muscle groups: Quadriceps, Hamstrings, Glutes
Secondary muscle groups: Calves, Abdominals, Spinal erectors

22

BASE

REVERSE LUNGE

23

INTERMEDIATE

WALKING LUNGE

24

INTERMEDIATE

SIDE LUNGE

Lunges create the opportunity to work your legs one at a time while also challenging your balance and core stability. Lunges can be done in many directions, but for this group of variations, we'll focus on reverse lunges, walking lunges, and side lunges. They all strengthen your quads, hamstrings, and glutes, giving you powerful, toned upper legs.

22 / REVERSE LUNGE

The reverse lunge is the simplest of the lunges because it doesn't require you to shift your base of support. As with the squat variations above, the working leg remains stationary throughout the entire movement of the reverse lunge, so your body has an easier time accommodating to the shift in your center of gravity that happens as the nonworking side moves backward. It's a great place to start building control of single-leg function and stabilization. Just make sure your shin and knee pass directly over your midfoot without causing your foot to turn out (see proper form for this shown in illustration B on page 93.) Your knee can come out over your toes as long as your weight stays evenly distributed across your foot.

GOAL: 20 repetitions on each side

1 Stand upright with your feet together. Ⓐ Slowly lift your left leg and step backward while at the same time bending your right knee to lower yourself toward the ground. You should be moving toward a half-kneeling position with your weight mainly on your standing (right) leg. Ⓑ

2 As the knee of your left leg approaches the ground, drive through your right leg and return to the starting position. Ⓐ

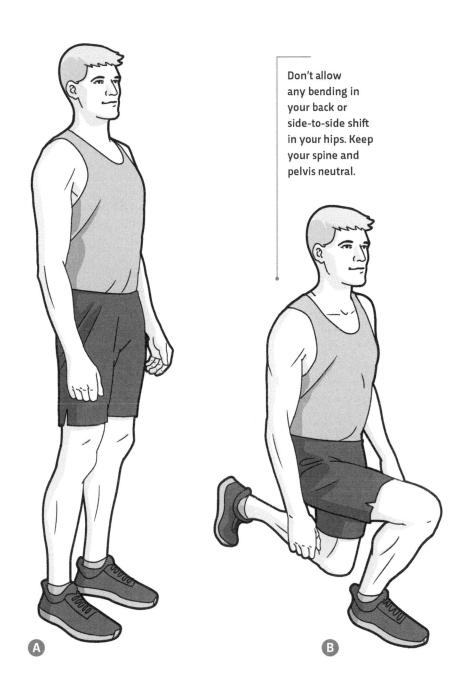

Don't allow any bending in your back or side-to-side shift in your hips. Keep your spine and pelvis neutral.

A

B

23 / WALKING LUNGE

This is one of the most functional variations of the lunge because it mimics and exaggerates a motion we do every day: walking. In this exercise you'll alternate lunging legs and travel across an open area. This lunge does involve changing your center of gravity and your base of support as you move, which makes it harder than the reverse lunge (22). Again, make sure your shin and knee pass directly over your midfoot and your weight is evenly distributed across your foot.

GOAL: 20 repetitions on each side

1 Stand upright with your feet together. **A** Step forward with one leg and slowly drop yourself toward a half-kneeling position. **B**

----

2 As your back knee approaches the ground, drive up through the front leg and return to the standing position you started in—except now you've traveled a few feet forward. **C**

----

3 Repeat, stepping forward with your other leg. **D**

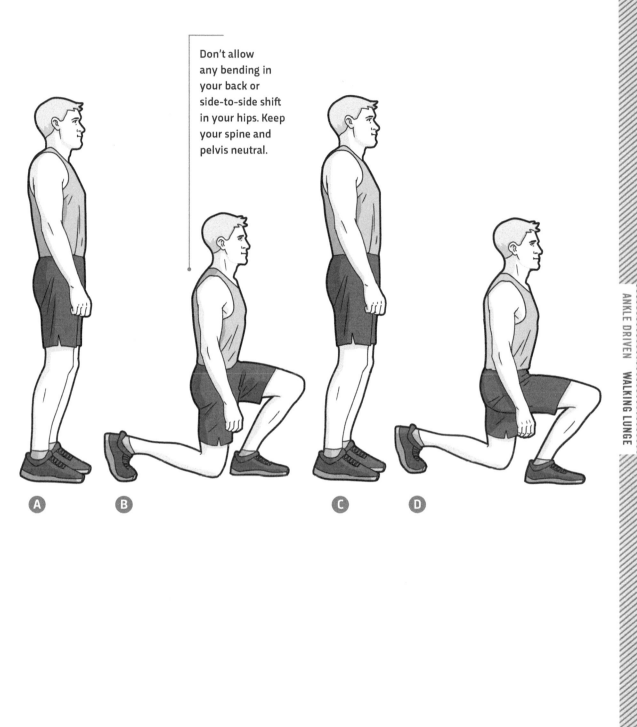

Don't allow
any bending in
your back or
side-to-side shift
in your hips. Keep
your spine and
pelvis neutral.

A   B   C   D

24 / SIDE LUNGE

In this variation, you step directly out to one side, dropping into a side lunge while maintaining a locked knee and planted foot on the trailing leg. You challenge the flexibility of the muscles that squeeze your thighs together as well as your stretch reflex as you push off the lunging side and pull yourself back to standing. You also develop your hip stabilization as you keep your hip, knee, and ankle in line with one another despite the sideways momentum as you drop into your lunge. As with all lunge variations, make sure your shin and knee pass directly over your midfoot and that your weight is evenly distributed across your foot.

GOAL: 20 repetitions on each side

1 Start with your feet together in a standing position. Step straight out to one side as far as you can, dropping into a lunge. Keep the trailing leg straight, the sole of your foot planted on the ground. **A**

2 As the thigh of the lunging leg gets close to being parallel with the floor, push through that midfoot and start momentum back toward your starting position.

3 Transfer your weight to the trailing leg as you rise and use your inner thigh to finish your return to a standing position. Repeat, stepping to the side with your other leg.

Don't allow any bending in your back or side-to-side shift in your hips. Keep your spine and pelvis neutral.

You can add a jumping (explosive) component to bodyweight staples like squats and lunges to ramp up the challenge. Just make sure you can perform the basic versions safely before you let your feet leave the ground between reps.

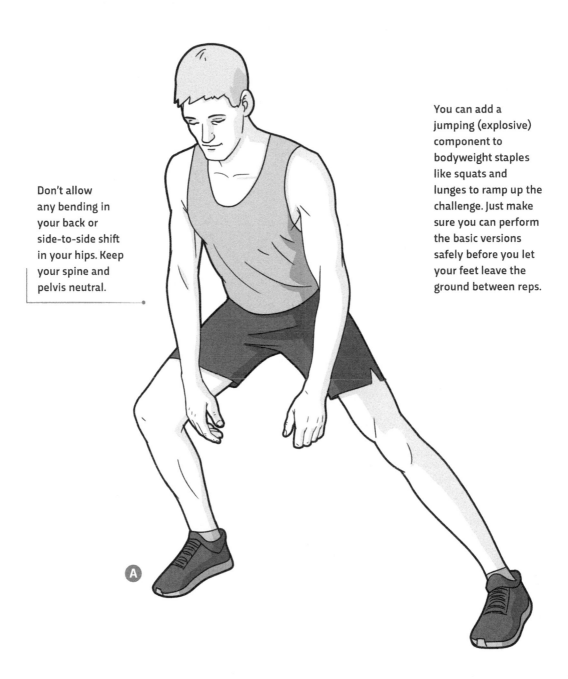

STEP-UP

Primary muscle groups: Quadriceps, Hamstrings, Glutes
Secondary muscle groups: Calves, Spinal erectors, Abdominals

25

BASE

FORWARD
STEP-UP

26

INTERMEDIATE

TRANSVERSE
STEP-UP

27

INTERMEDIATE

FORWARD
STEP-DOWN

The step-up is another classic functional exercise because it imitates one of the main ways we change our elevation in everyday life: climbing stairs. These step-up variations all require a sturdy step, bench, or retaining wall close to knee height, and they'll all help strengthen your quads, glutes, and hamstrings. Like lunges, step-ups can be done in several directions. Here you'll focus on a forward step-up, a transverse step-up, and a forward step-down.

25 / FORWARD STEP-UP

The forward step-up involves a large range of ankle dorsiflexion, where you bend at the ankle, moving your shin forward over the top of your foot. That means it's extra important that your shin and knee pass straight over the middle of your foot and that your foot is not turned out. As your weight shifts forward, you'll feel your upper body start to lean forward and your hips push backward to accommodate a stiff ankle. Try not to let that happen. You may also notice your hip shifting sideways, which is another compensation you want to avoid. In this exercise you'll step up and lower yourself repeatedly with the same leg until you reach your desired repetitions before switching to the other side. Keep your spine neutral and strive for good control of your ankle and foot.

GOAL: **The greater range of motion you develop in your ankle joints, the more control you'll have over your ankle and foot. When you can do 20 repetitions on each side, you're ready for the Transverse Step-Up (26).**

1 Stand roughly 12 inches from your chosen step. Raise one leg and place that foot flat on top of the step. **A** Find the right amount of bend in your ankle joint to keep the hip, knee, and ankle in line with each other.

----

2 Keeping your spine neutral, drive up through your high leg and bring yourself to a standing position on top of the step. **B**

----

3 With the same working leg, slowly lower yourself back to the starting position. **A**

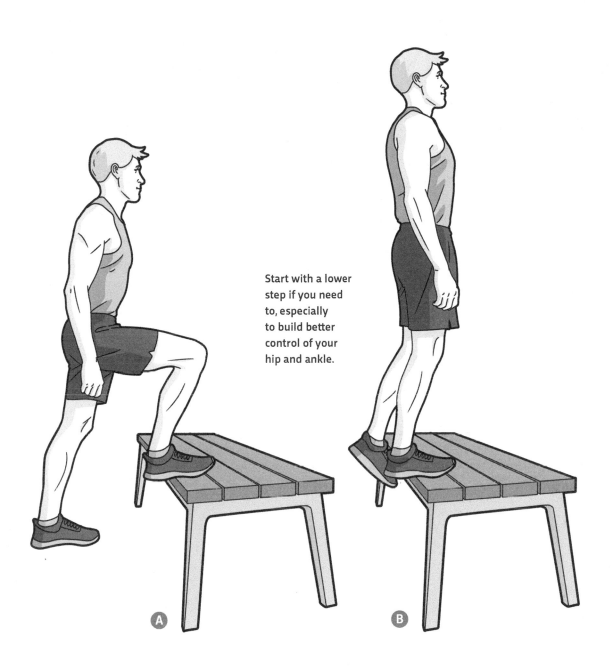

Start with a lower
step if you need
to, especially
to build better
control of your
hip and ankle.

A

B

26 / TRANSVERSE STEP-UP

This variation is similar to the forward step-up (25), but at first, you turn 45 degrees from the step, turning your body at your hip—not your spine—as you make your step up and then again as you reverse the motion. In addition to working your upper legs, this *transverse*, or "crosswise," aspect forces your hips to stabilize through internal and external rotation. As with the forward step-up, keep your spine neutral.

GOAL: Facing sideways to the step with your foot at 90 degrees.
20 repetitions on each side

1 Stand roughly 12 inches from your chosen step, with your body turned away from the step at 45 degrees, and your foot on the step, also at 45 degrees. **A**

----

2 Press up evenly through the foot on the step, lifting your body while simultaneously rotating your hip **B** and coming to rest on the top of the step with your feet together.

----

3 Return to your starting position by reversing the movement **C** and stepping down while turning out. **A**

You can start with a lower step and a smaller rotational angle. The goal is to turn sideways to the step, and step up at 90 degrees.

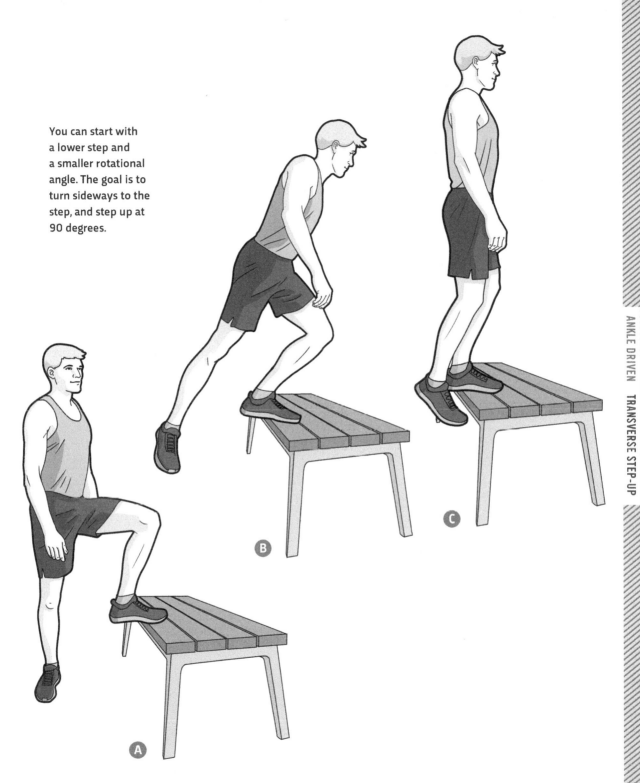

27 / FORWARD STEP-DOWN

Although here you'll step down instead of up, you're still working your upper legs and glutes. You're also working your knees. In fact, this exercise can put excessive pressure on your knees, especially if you lack proper flexibility in your hips and ankles, so please perform it with caution, and stop if it causes knee pain or if you have a known issue that might be subject to injury. Start by stepping down from something the height of a curb, then gradually increase to something mid-shin height if you want more difficulty. Pay close attention to your ankle, and prevent the predictable compensation: your foot turning out. This is especially important on the back leg during the second half of the motion as you return to the starting position.

GOAL: **Work on landing softly with your stepping leg, making as little noise as possible. Aim to do 10 repetitions on each side.**

1 Stand on a curb or a step about 4 to 8 inches high with your toes at its edge. Ⓐ

2 Slowly step forward, controlling your descent with the back leg Ⓑ until the forward leg makes contact with the ground on the lower level and bends to absorb the shock.

3 Descend into your forward leg until the knee of your back leg reaches the height of the curb or step. Ⓒ

4 Drive off the midfoot of your front leg, springing off the ground and finishing your momentum by returning your back leg to its starting position. Ⓐ

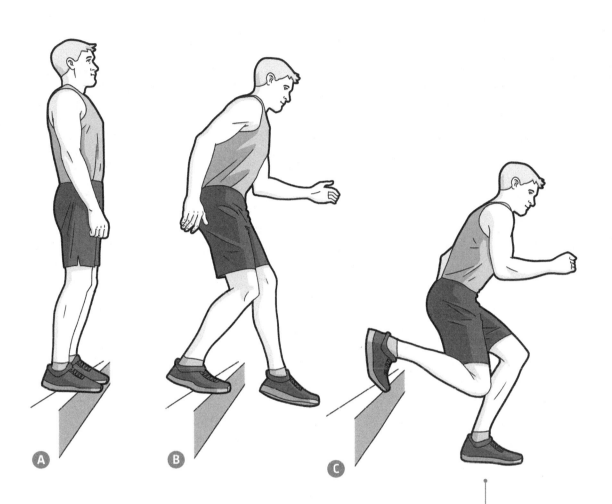

Focus on the deceleration of the front leg as you step off the curb and then explode back to the start position.

JUMP

Primary muscle groups: Quadriceps, Hamstrings, Glutes
Secondary muscle groups: Calves, Abdominals, Spinal erectors

28
BASE

FLOOR JUMP

29
INTERMEDIATE

BOX JUMP

30
ADVANCED

ONE LEG POWER JUMP

Jumps are a great way to build the explosive power of your legs and get your heart rate up, but don't do them until you can squat comfortably without your knees turning inward. Your ankles, knees, and hips should remain in line with each other throughout the entire jump and should be strong enough to slowly lower your body weight as you land. Here you'll start with a stationary floor jump straight up in the air, then progress to a box jump and, for a real challenge, a one-leg power jump from a staggered stance with the working leg up on a step.

28 / FLOOR JUMP

The floor jump is a stationary jump without equipment. You jump as high as you can straight up in the air. As you land, you comfortably absorb the shock with your feet closer together and then take a small hop back and drop back into a three-quarter squat for the next rep. As you get better, you can try landing directly back in the three-quarter squat and immediately starting the next rep without any pause.

GOAL: Slowly eliminate the regressed landing until you can land directly in the three-quarters squat and rapidly repeat the motion. When you can do 20 repetitions with that squat landing, you're ready to try Box Jumps (29).

1 Stand with your feet shoulder-width apart. Squat to about three-quarters depth **A** and spring up, jumping just a few inches forward and landing upright. **B** Remember to keep your ankles, knees, and hips in line the whole time.

2 Hop backward a few inches, absorbing the shock of the landing with a three-quarters squat. **C**

3 Repeat the jump sequence, traveling slightly forward during the jump and slightly backward during the return.

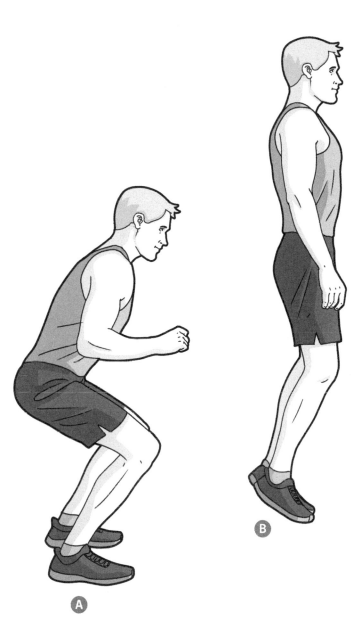

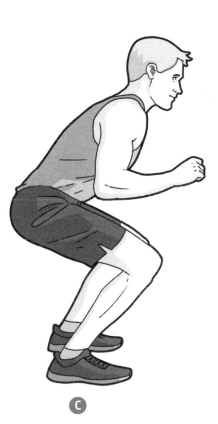

Tuck your knees up toward your chest during the jump to test your wind even more.

A

B

C

29 / BOX JUMP

Box jumps are like floor jumps (28), except instead of landing back on the floor, you jump up onto a step, box, or other elevated surface. They allow you to train only the explosive phase of movement associated with jumping without worrying as much about shock absorption. Jumping onto an elevated level is more difficult, but it puts much less stress on your joints, so you can do more reps without fear of injury. It can be a little unnerving to jump to another surface, so proceed with caution. When you step back down off the step at the end of the jump, alternate the leg you use so each leg gets similar work. And as with any jump, don't forget to maintain functional alignment throughout.

GOAL: 20 repetitions

1 Stand with your feet shoulder-width apart about 12 inches in front of a knee-high step or other elevated surface.

2 Drop into a three-quarters squat. **A** Quickly spring up and forward as high as you can, landing on top of the step. **B**

3 Drive up through your legs to a standing position on top of the step. **C** Step backward off the step as you would during the second half of a forward step-up (25), alternating the working leg with each repetition.

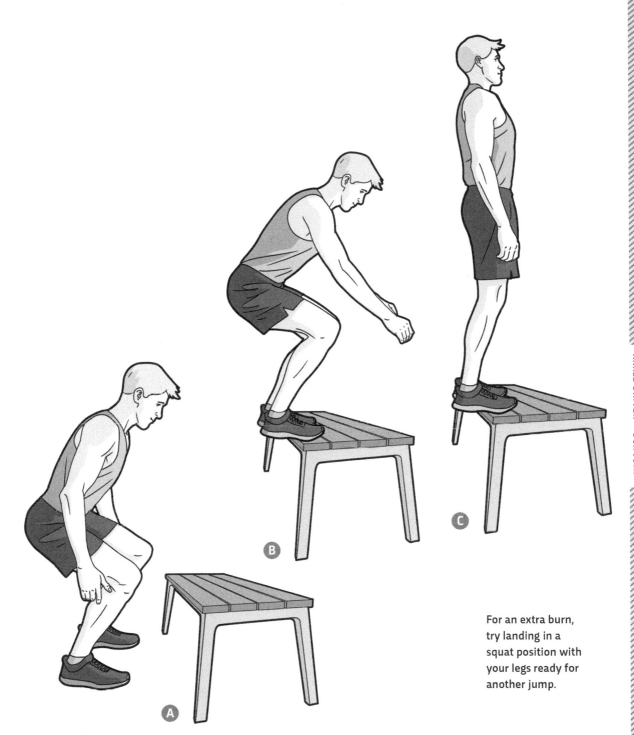

A

B

C

For an extra burn, try landing in a squat position with your legs ready for another jump.

30 / ONE LEG POWER JUMP

Ready to jump with one leg? Here you use a step like you did with the box jump (29) in order to soften your landing and allow for more rapid repetitions. Those rapid reps are great for building not just leg strength but also cardiovascular efficiency.

GOAL: Work toward maintaining 4 inches or more of vertical jump through every repetition. Aim to do 20 repetitions on each side.

1 Stand in front of your step with one foot up on the step and the other on ground level. (A)

2 Jump up, pressing off the foot on the step to jump as high as you can. (B)

3 Land on that same leg, still on the step, and slowly lower your weight as the other leg lands back on the ground in its original position. (A)

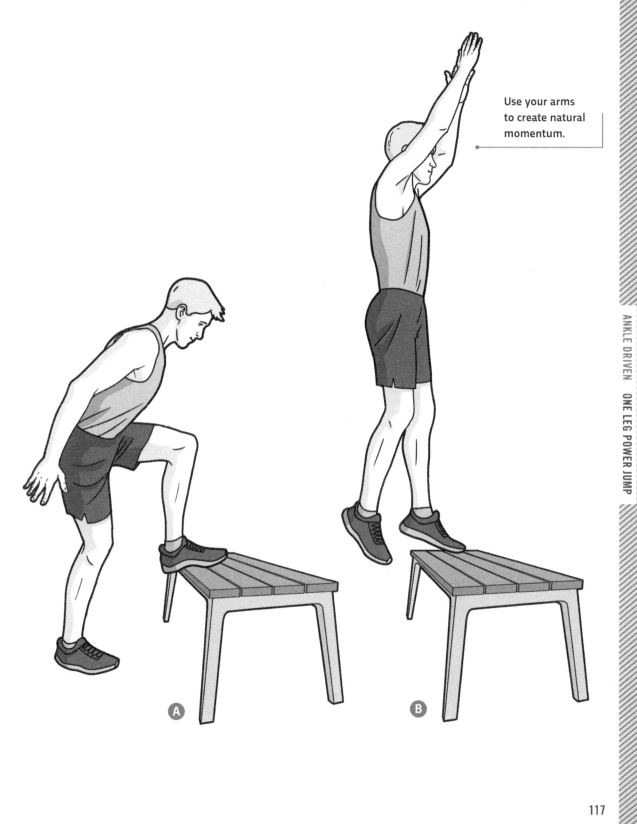

Use your arms to create natural momentum.

A

B

DYNAMIC JUMP

Primary muscle groups: Quadriceps, Hamstrings, Glutes
Secondary muscle groups: Calves, Abdominals, Spinal erectors

31

BASE

ICE SKATER

32

INTERMEDIATE

BROAD JUMP

33

ADVANCED

POWER BOUND

A jump is classified as *dynamic* when it involves a large shift in your center of gravity and direction. This makes the jumps much more difficult for your nervous system to handle, because your brain has to figure out how to keep your balance and activate different muscles accordingly. Dynamic jumps help train your ankles, hips, core, and leg muscles to react to the demands put on them, while still providing stability.

31 / ICE SKATER

Ice skaters are dynamic jumps that mimic the side-to-side motions you make when cutting direction on a playing field or court. Your goal is to cover as much horizontal distance as you can with each jump, not to jump high up into the air. This is another great exercise for increasing your heart rate, and like the side lunge (24), it improves your hip stabilization as you try to keep your knee in line with your ankle and hip.

GOAL: **Work toward a stride length of half your height. So if you're 6 feet tall, aim to jump 3 feet to the side.**

1 Stand with your feet together and your knees slightly bent. Hop out to your right as far as you can, landing on your right foot (A), which should face straight forward as you land. Allow your knee to bend as you absorb the shock. Let your left leg pass behind your right, and your arms cross your body, to help prep for the next jump.

- -

2 Immediately push off your right foot and hop in the other direction, landing on your left foot. (B) Continue alternating between feet, trying to cover as much horizontal ground as possible.

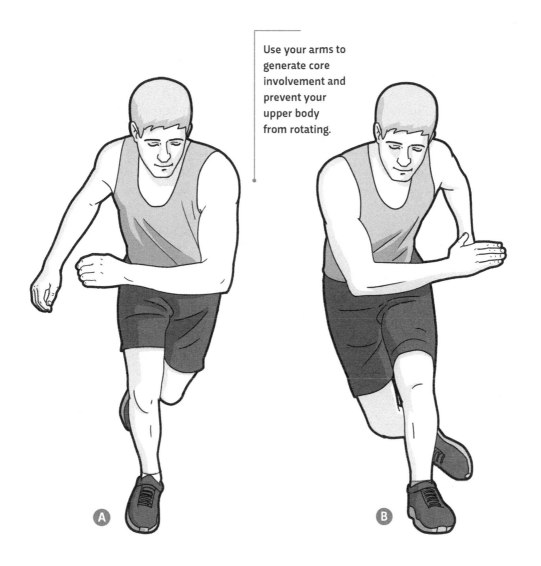

Use your arms to generate core involvement and prevent your upper body from rotating.

A

B

32 / BROAD JUMP

The broad jump is another explosive movement that allows you to take off and land on the same surface. Like the ice skater (31), the broad jump tries to cover as much horizontal distance as possible, but this time you jump forward instead of to the side. Both your feet should take off together and land together, making as little noise as possible. Make sure your hips, knees, and ankles stay in line. Do not allow your knees to collapse inward during take-off or landing.

GOAL: You want to reposition your feet as minimally as possible between jumps. **Work up to doing 20 repetitions.**

1 Stand with your feet shoulder-width apart. Drop into a three-quarters squat, **A** then spring forward, going for distance, not height. **B**

2 Land with both feet in another three-quarters squat. **A**

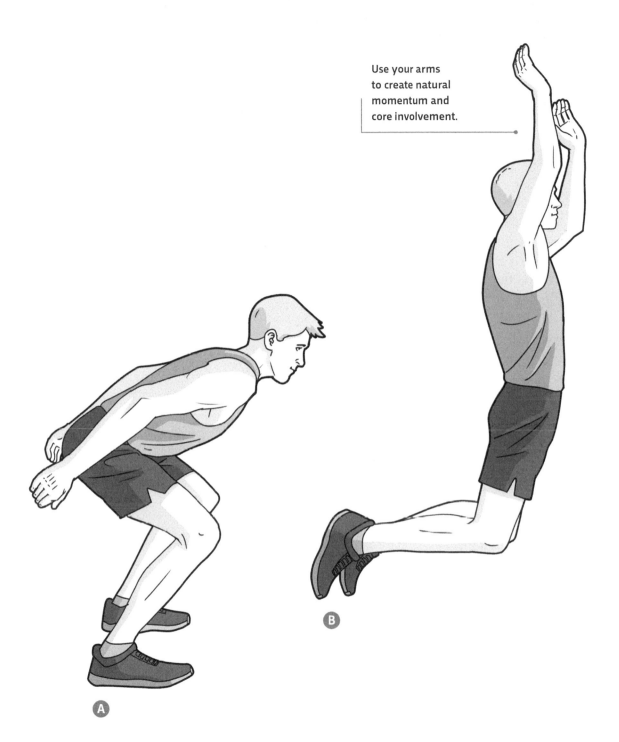

Use your arms
to create natural
momentum and
core involvement.

A

B

33 / POWER BOUND

Power bounds are essentially adult-size skips that you use to travel as far as you possibly can. Again, distance will be your priority here, so you'll need some space for this exercise. If you need to do it in circles to fit inside a certain area, go ahead, but make sure you switch directions with each set.

GOAL: Work toward a stride length of three-quarters of your height. So if you're 6 feet tall, you should be jumping about 4.5 feet forward. Aim to do 20 repetitions on each side.

1 Start in a staggered stance, aligning the toes of your back foot with the heel of your front foot, with the arm that's on the same side as your back foot forward. **A**

----

2 Drive your forward arm back and your backward arm forward as you leap from your forward leg as far as you can, landing on that same leg. **B**

----

3 When you land, quickly take a step with the other leg, landing in a staggered stance so that you're ready to repeat the motion on the other side.

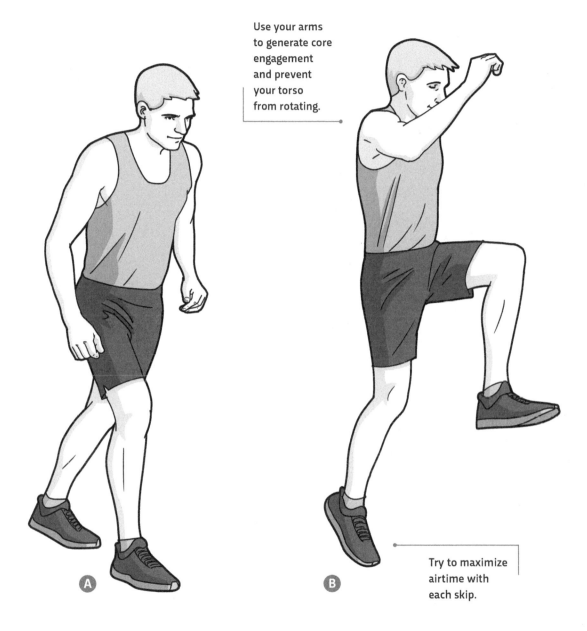

Use your arms to generate core engagement and prevent your torso from rotating.

Try to maximize airtime with each skip.

A

B

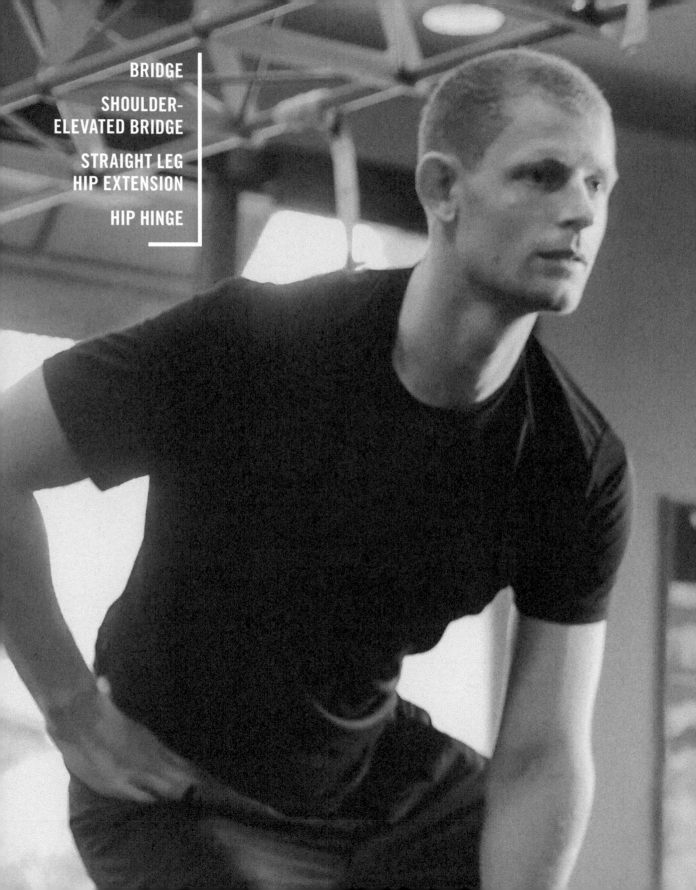

BRIDGE

SHOULDER-
ELEVATED BRIDGE

STRAIGHT LEG
HIP EXTENSION

HIP HINGE

A movement can be described as *hip-driven* when the predominant action involves the thigh bone moving within the pelvis. The lower back should resist both flexion and extension, remaining neutral through all movements. In standing hip-driven exercises, the shin bone (tibia) remains vertical, while in floor exercises, the knee stays mostly static, making your glutes and

HIP
DRIVEN

hamstrings do the majority of the work of moving your hips. Control of this area is extremely important, because the tilt of your pelvis has a huge effect on the stability and safety of your highly vulnerable lower spine, as well as your abdominals' ability to engage properly. If you don't develop healthy movement patterns in your hips, you're likely to end up with lower-back pain. The exercises in this chapter will help you develop those patterns so you can build your core and legs without injuring yourself.

BRIDGE

Primary muscle groups: Glutes, Hamstrings
Secondary muscle group: Abdominals

34
BASE

**FLOOR
BRIDGE**

35
INTERMEDIATE

**ONE LEG
FLOOR
BRIDGE**

36
ADVANCED

**ELEVATED
BRIDGE**

The most basic of the hip-driven exercises are the bridges. You do them from a supine position (lying on your back) with your knees in a relatively fixed position so that most of the movement comes from your hips. It's easy to accidentally start using your lower back to help generate some of the motion, so pay close attention to your pelvic tilt and don't let it change throughout the entire exercise. These exercises target hip extensors, like the glutes and hamstrings for movement, and core muscles for stabilization. The three variations covered here are the basic floor bridge, the one leg floor bridge, and the elevated bridge.

34 / FLOOR BRIDGE

The basic floor bridge puts your body in a stable position, leaving your nervous system available to fully focus on the task at hand instead of using it to fight gravity and stay balanced. It's a great way to learn the fundamentals of hip-driven movements: Once you've figured out how to work your pelvis and femur together properly while restricting motion in your lower back, you'll be able to use that proper form for all hip-driven exercises. The basic floor bridge uses a relatively small range of motion, but it's a great bodyweight exercise and learning opportunity.

GOAL: You'll know you've mastered the basic floor bridge when you can perform the motion with no spinal movement. Aim to do 20 perfect repetitions before progressing to the One Leg Floor Bridge (35).

1 Lie on your back with your knees bent and your feet on the ground. Your heels should be just within reach of your fingertips. Ⓐ

----

2 Making sure your lower spine is neutral, drive up through your heels, pushing your pelvis up toward the sky. Ⓑ

----

3 Once your hips are fully extended, slowly return to the starting position. Ⓐ

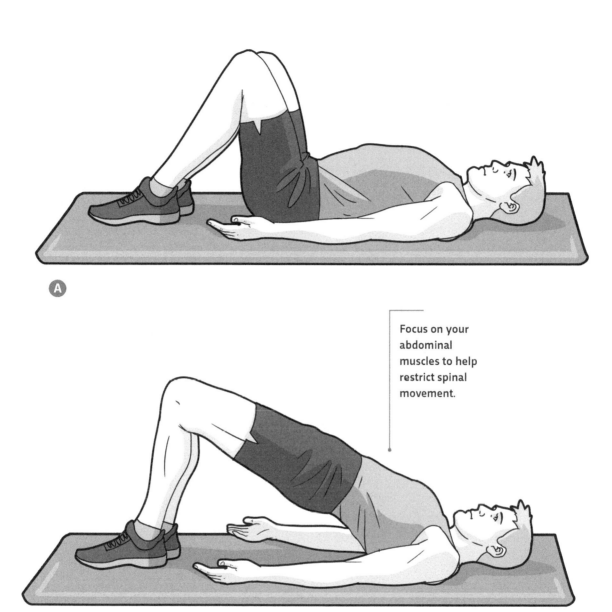

Focus on your abdominal muscles to help restrict spinal movement.

Think of your shoulders as the point of rotation on the ground.

35 / ONE LEG FLOOR BRIDGE

The one leg floor bridge will challenge the strength and stability of your hip muscles on one side of your body, as well as your ability to extend one hip while the other is bending. This is a movement pattern most people have lost in modern-day life, so you'll probably need to retrain yourself to do it. You should not attempt this variation until you're proficient with the basic floor bridge (34) and can restrict the movement in your spine while allowing your femur and pelvis to work together in proper alignment.

GOAL: Eventually you should be able to fully extend the working hip while your hips remain parallel with ground. Work toward doing 20 repetitions on each side.

1 Lie on your back with your knees bent and your feet on the ground. Your heels should be just within reach of your fingertips. Grab one knee, and pull it up toward your chest. **A**

----

2 Making sure your lower spine is neutral, drive up through the heel that's still on the floor, pushing your pelvis toward the sky and making sure not to rotate your hips in either direction. **A**

----

3 Once your down hip is fully extended, slowly return to the starting position.

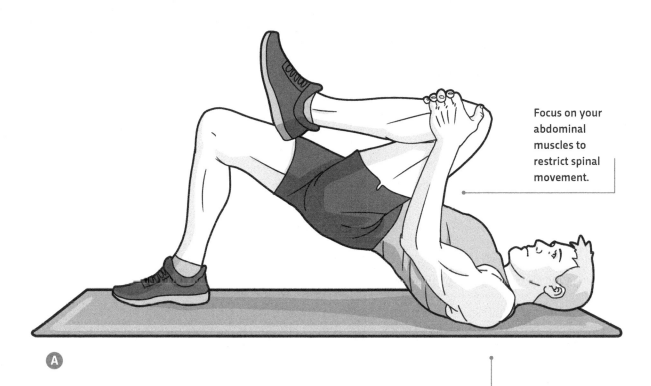

Focus on your abdominal muscles to restrict spinal movement.

Think of your shoulders as the point of rotation on the ground.

A

36 / ELEVATED BRIDGE

In this variation, you elevate your feet on a small step to allow your hips a slightly larger range of motion. The same rules about unwanted spinal movement apply: Your femur and pelvis should work together in proper alignment without moving your spine. Make sure you finish the elevated bridge with your pelvis neutral, not stuck in a forward tilt with your lower back arched.

GOAL: 20 repetitions

1 Lie on your back with your knees bent and your feet on a small step about curb height (4 to 8 inches high). Your heels should be just within reach of your fingertips. **A**

----

2 Making sure your lower spine is neutral, drive up through your heels, pushing your pelvis toward the sky. **B**

----

3 Once your hips are fully extended, slowly return to the starting position. **A**

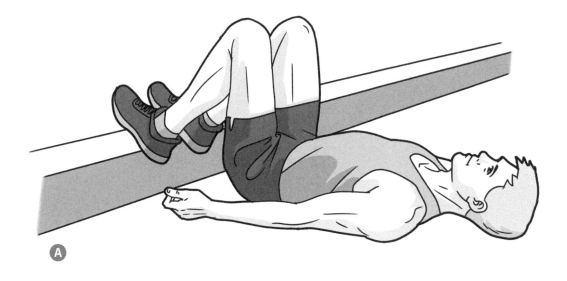

A

For an extra challenge, try doing the elevated bridge with only one leg at a time.

Hold the contraction for up to seven seconds for maximum muscle activation.

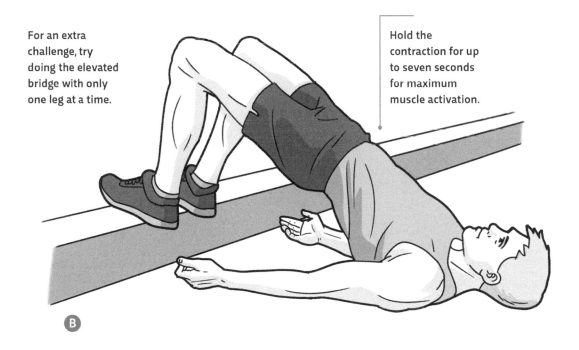

B

SHOULDER-ELEVATED BRIDGE

Primary muscle groups: Glutes, Hamstrings
Secondary muscle groups: Abdominals, Deltoids

37

BASE

SHOULDER-ELEVATED BRIDGE

38

INTERMEDIATE

ONE LEG SHOULDER-ELEVATED BRIDGE

39

INTERMEDIATE

ONE ARM SHOULDER-ELEVATED BRIDGE

In this variation on the bridge, elevating your shoulders gives your hips a larger range of motion. To elevate your shoulders, place your hands on the ground with your arms rotated outward so the insides of your elbows are pointing down toward your hips. You can also place your shoulders on a knee-height step or bench if one is available, but performing this movement from your hands provides a good dynamic stretch through your biceps and the front of your shoulders if you can handle it. It's important to master control of your lumbo-pelvic hip complex (the area of your body comprising the hip joint, lower spine, and pelvis) before attempting these variations. All the movement must be in the hips and shoulders—not the spine.

37 / SHOULDER-ELEVATED BRIDGE

The basic shoulder-elevated bridge uses both hands and both legs. You work your glutes and hamstrings by extending your hips to bring yourself up into a tabletop position, then returning to your resting position with your hips on the ground. Make sure your spine maintains its neutral relationship with your pelvis and that you don't recruit it to help with the motion. If this exercise is too painful on your shoulders, use a step or bench to elevate your shoulders instead of holding yourself up with your hands.

GOAL: Once you can do 20 repetitions with your spine completely neutral, you're ready to try the One Leg Shoulder-Elevated Bridge (38).

1 Start by sitting on the ground with your knees bent and your feet flat on the floor in front of you. Place your hands on the ground with your fingertips pointing behind you. **A**

2 Keeping your chest tall and your spine neutral, drive up through both heels and fully extend your hips, bringing your body into a tabletop position. **B**

3 Using your abdominals to keep your lower spine and pelvis in a neutral position, slowly lower your body back to its starting position. **A**

Try to keep your head and neck in a neutral position.

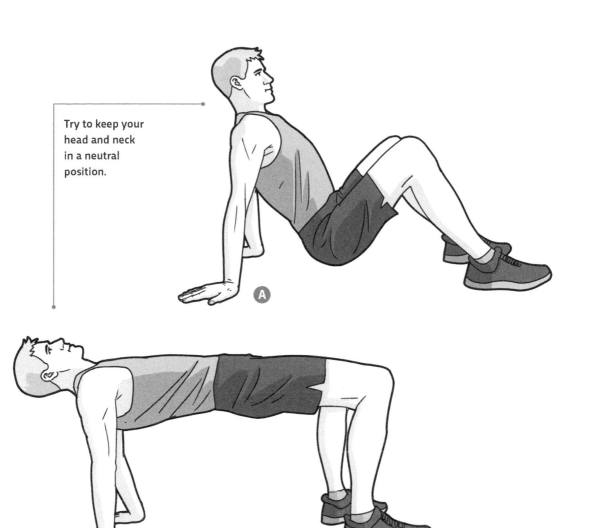

A

B

To reduce strain on your shoulders, try elevating them on a step or bench.

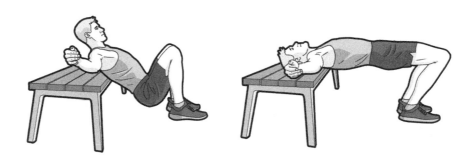

38 / ONE LEG SHOULDER-ELEVATED BRIDGE

This variation challenges one hip at a time. By lifting one leg, you greatly reduce your base of support for the exercise, which forces you to use your core and hip stabilizers to resist your body's natural tendency to rotate as compensation for the reduction in contact points.

GOAL: When you can do 20 repetitions on each side with your spine completely neutral, you're ready to move to the One Arm Shoulder-Elevated Bridge (39).

1 Start by sitting on the ground with your knees bent and your feet flat on the floor in front of you. Place your hands on the ground with your fingertips pointing behind you.

----

2 Keeping your chest tall and your spine neutral, straighten one knee, fixing that leg in an extended position. **A**

----

3 Drive up through the heel that's still on the floor and fully extend your hips, bringing your body into a three-legged tabletop position. **B**

----

4 Using your abdominals to keep your lower spine and pelvis in a neutral position, slowly lower your body back to its starting position.

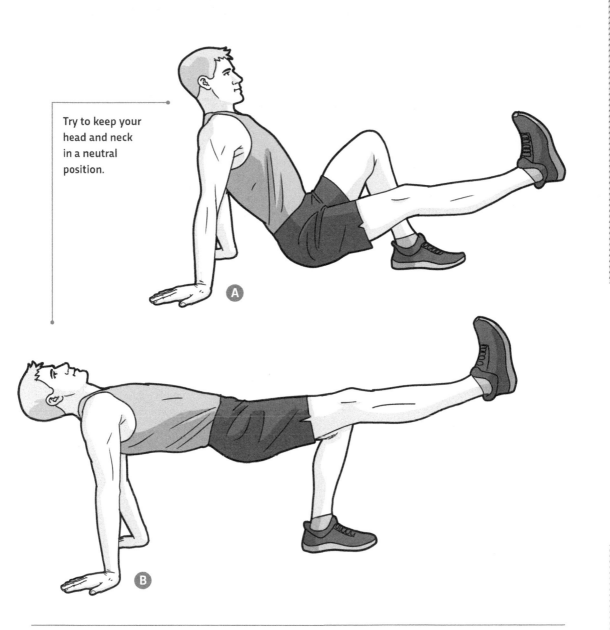

Try to keep your head and neck in a neutral position.

A

B

To reduce strain on your shoulders, try elevating them on a step or bench.

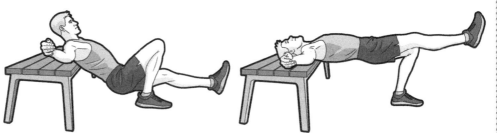

39 / ONE ARM SHOULDER-ELEVATED BRIDGE

The one arm shoulder-elevated bridge challenges your core stabilization from the top down rather than from the bottom up. It requires a great deal of shoulder mobility and stabilization, so don't attempt this variation if you have any tightness in your shoulders that causes pain or affects your ability to keep your upper spine straight.

GOAL: **Work toward doing 20 repetitions on each side without any rotation through your hips.**

1 Start by sitting on the ground with your knees bent and your feet flat on the floor in front of you. Place your hands on the ground with your fingertips pointing behind you.

----

2 Keeping your chest tall and your spine neutral, raise one hand off the ground and place it out to one side. **A**

----

3 Drive up through both heels and fully extend your hips, bringing your body into a three-legged tabletop position. **A**

----

4 Using your abdominals to keep your lower spine and pelvis in a neutral position, slowly lower your body back to its starting position.

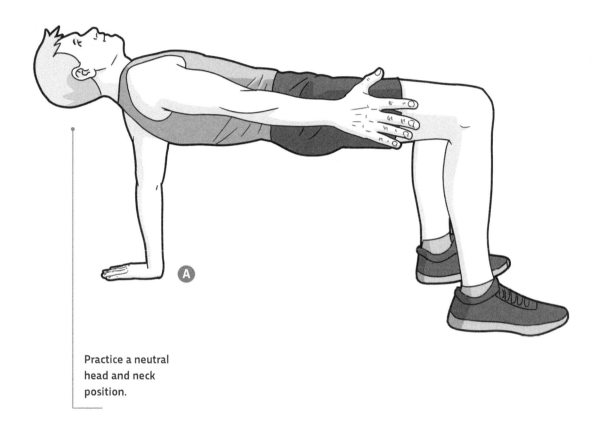

Practice a neutral
head and neck
position.

Ⓐ

STRAIGHT LEG HIP EXTENSION

Primary muscle group: Glutes
Secondary muscle group: Hamstrings

40
BASE

SIDE LYING LEG RAISE

41
INTERMEDIATE

QUADRUPED STRAIGHT TAP

42
ADVANCED

QUADRUPED OBLIQUE TAP

In these hip-driven movements, you focus on control of the hip joint alone, allowing no other joints to move at the same time. They can be done lying on your side or on all fours, and they all focus on extending the hips with the knee locked. This means you're using only the many fibers of the glutes to drive the motion, which is why straight leg hip extensions are a great way to strengthen and tone your backside. Here you'll start with a side lying leg raise to activate the stabilizing glute fibers, a chronically underactive muscle often responsible for collapsing your knees during ankle-driven movements. Then you'll move on to a variation that targets the meat of the glutes, and end with one that works the whole gluteal complex.

40 / SIDE LYING LEG RAISE

This exercise focuses on activating the gluteus medius, the stabilizing muscles of the hip. As you perform the motion, make sure your toes are pointed down toward the ground, and let your upper body lie flat on its side. Don't prop yourself up on your elbow—that only causes your spine to bend from side to side.

GOAL: 20 repetitions on each side

1 Lie flat on your side with your hips lined up vertically. Do not prop your upper body up on your elbow.

----

2 Point the toes of your top foot down toward the ground, and place your top hand on your abdominals to feel for any unwanted movement. **A**

----

3 While keeping your knee locked and toes pointed down, elevate your top foot as high as possible **B** without bending your spine from side to side to assist in the motion.

----

4 Once your foot is as high as it can go, slowly return it to its starting position. **A**

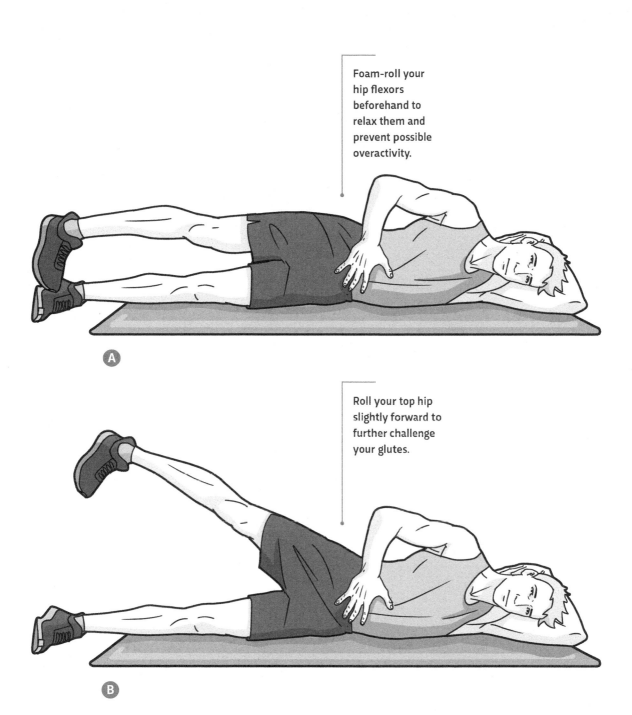

Foam-roll your hip flexors beforehand to relax them and prevent possible overactivity.

Roll your top hip slightly forward to further challenge your glutes.

A

B

41 / QUADRUPED STRAIGHT TAP

Done on all fours (*quadruped*), this variation challenges the bulk of the glutes to perform isolated hip extensions. It's important to activate your abdominals to prevent any unwanted lower-spine extension. Keep your knee locked and your quad active to inhibit hamstring function and leave your glutes fully responsible for creating the motion. If your hip flexors are tight, contracting your glutes will be difficult. If that's the case, focus more on mobility work during your cooldowns. Spend more time in the half-kneeling position to train your hip flexors to get longer.

GOAL: As you get stronger, you can try to get your leg slightly higher than parallel with your spine (but still in a neutral position). Work up to doing 20 repetitions on each side.

1 Start on all fours with your hands directly below your shoulders and your knees directly below your hips.

----

2 Straighten one leg out behind you, leaving just the toes in contact with the ground.

----

3 While keeping your quad tight to maintain a locked knee **A**, squeeze your glutes to raise your back leg up as high as you can without using your low back. **B** Be sure to use your abdominals to prevent your lower spine from assisting in the leg raise.

----

4 Slowly lower your leg to the ground, lightly tapping your toes on the ground before going straight into the next rep.

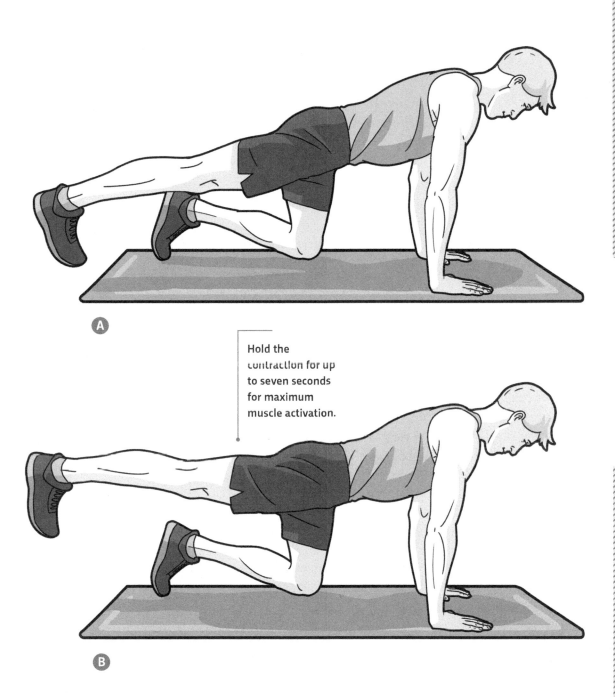

Hold the contraction for up to seven seconds for maximum muscle activation.

A

B

42 / QUADRUPED OBLIQUE TAP

In this variation, you challenge your hip extension in three positions: abducted (away from your body's midline), adducted (toward your body's midline), and neutral. Try to keep your toes pointed directly downward as you do each tap (to the outside, straight back, and to the far side of the opposite leg). A tap in each position counts as one repetition. Stabilizing your lower spine and your pelvis is crucial to performing this exercise correctly.

GOAL: Work toward doing 21 repetitions (7 cycles of 3 taps in different directions) on each side.

1 Start on all fours with your hands directly below your shoulders and your knees directly below your hips. Straighten your right leg out behind you, leaving just the toes in contact with the ground. Ⓐ

2 While keeping your quad tight to maintain a locked knee, squeeze your glutes to raise your right leg up as high as you can. Then, slowly lower your leg to its starting position, lightly tapping your toes on the ground.

3 On the next rep, instead of tapping your toes straight back down again, tap the ground slightly to your right. On the rep after that, tap the ground slightly to the left of your left leg. Ⓑ

4 Continue tapping in cycles of three: once straight back, once slightly to the outside of the active leg, and once slightly to the outside of the stationary leg.

5 Switch to your left leg and repeat.

Before you start, stretch your hips by rotating them inward and outward. You'll be able to move your leg farther and challenge more muscle fiber.

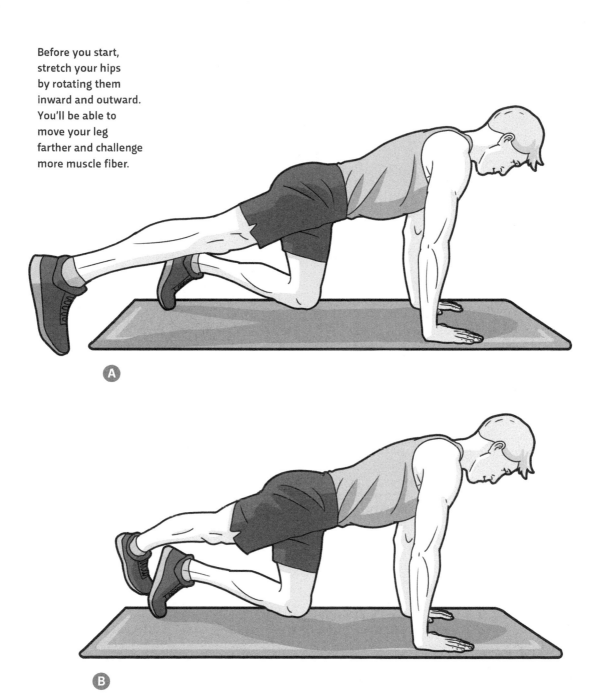

A

B

HIP HINGE

Primary muscle groups: Glutes, Hamstrings
Secondary muscle groups: Spinal erectors, Abdominals

43

BASE

TWO LEG HIP HINGE

44

INTERMEDIATE

STAGGERED HIP HINGE

45

ADVANCED

ONE LEG HIP HINGE

The hip hinge is the most functional of the hip-driven exercises because it mimics a movement most of us use multiple times a day: bending over. The hip-hinge variations here require you to use your motor control to restrict motion in your spine while still allowing motion in your hips. They're all forward-bending patterns that test your hips' full range of motion and reinforce healthy movement habits. Keep in mind that a healthy bending pattern has you push your hips and butt backward as you bend. And because this is a hip-driven activity, not an ankle-driven one, try to restrict the bending of your ankle.

43 / TWO LEG HIP HINGE

The hip hinge is an extremely important human movement pattern. It forms the foundation for all sorts of lower-body movements, from bending over to pick up the keys you dropped to performing flawless burpees. The idea is to lower your upper body while keeping your knees positioned over your ankles and not flexing your spine at all. You can soften your knees to allow your hips to move backward into the posterior weight shift that is necessary for a healthy bend, but don't let your knees come forward.

GOAL: When you can do 20 repetitions while keeping your spine perfectly neutral and stable, you're ready to try the Staggered Hip Hinge (44).

1 Stand with the insteps of your feet shoulder-width apart, your arms down at your sides.

----

2 Soften your knees and shift your weight backward as you lower your torso forward toward the ground, **A** maintaining a neutral spine the whole time.

----

3 Keep bending until you feel a stretch in your hamstrings or your spine becomes parallel to the ground, then squeeze your glutes and return to your starting position.

To increase
difficulty, hold
your arms static
overhead while
performing
the motion.

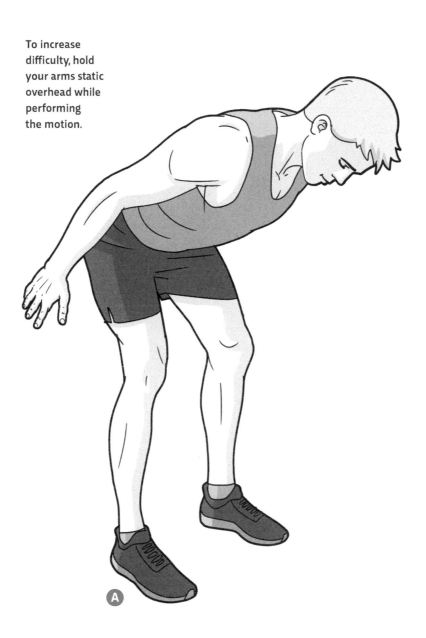

44 / STAGGERED HIP HINGE

This variation works on hip stability one leg at a time. Your other leg helps you balance but doesn't really do any work. Your feet are much closer together than they were for the basic two leg hip hinge (43), and they're staggered, with the back foot up on its toes. Be careful not to rotate the working hip outward—this is caused by lack of activity of your hip stabilizers. By keeping your hips parallel with the ground, you'll train your stabilizers to fire earlier and work in cooperation with the rest of your glutes.

GOAL: **20 repetitions on each side without rotating your working hip outward at all**

1 Stand with your feet hip-width apart and slightly staggered—one foot in front of the other, aligning the toes of the back foot with the heel of the front foot. Keep the front foot flat on the ground, but lift the heel of the back foot.

----

2 Soften your knees and shift your weight backward as you lower your torso forward toward the ground. **A** Maintain a neutral spine, and be careful not to rotate out through your hips.

----

3 Keep bending until you feel a stretch in your working hamstring or your spine becomes parallel to the ground. Squeeze your working leg's glutes, and return to the starting position.

To increase
difficulty, hold
your arms static
overhead while
performing
the motion.

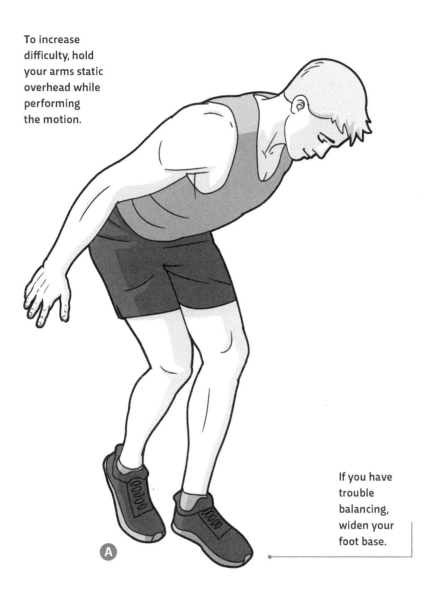

A

If you have
trouble
balancing,
widen your
foot base.

45 / ONE LEG HIP HINGE

The one leg hip hinge is just what it sounds like—a hip hinge performed on one leg—and it's the ultimate functional hip-driven bodyweight movement. It challenges balance, hip stability, and core stability as well as controlled mobility of the hip joint. It's the last step in the hip-hinge progressions, and everyone should master it. Shifting your center of gravity over such a small base of support demonstrates great strength and balance control. Make sure your hips stay square with the ground and aren't rotating outward because of weak stabilizers. Keep an eye on the toes of your nonworking leg: If they start to point outward, that's a good indicator that your hips are rotating outward. Activate the glutes of the nonworking leg to help stabilize the motion.

GOAL: 20 repetitions on each side without rotating your working hip outward at all

1 Stand with your feet hip-width apart and slightly staggered, one foot in front of the other, aligning the toes of the back foot with the heel of the front foot. Keep the front foot flat on the ground, but lift the heel of the back foot.

2 Soften your knees and shift your weight backward as you lower your torso forward toward the ground and extend your back leg out behind you. **A** Maintain a neutral spine, and be careful not to rotate through your hips.

3 Keep bending until you feel a stretch in your working hamstring or your spine becomes parallel to the ground. Squeeze your working leg's glutes, and return to the starting position.

To increase difficulty, hold your arms static overhead while performing the motion.

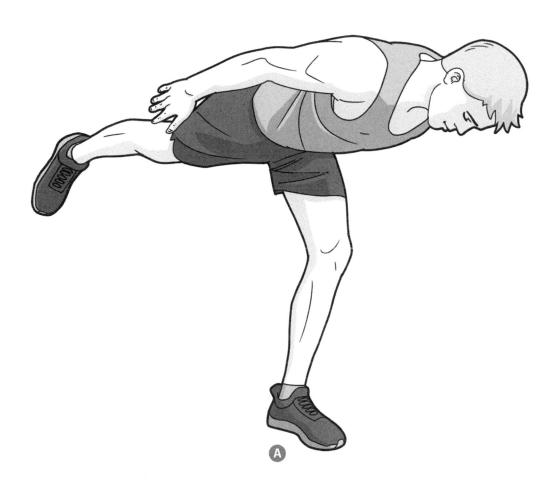

A

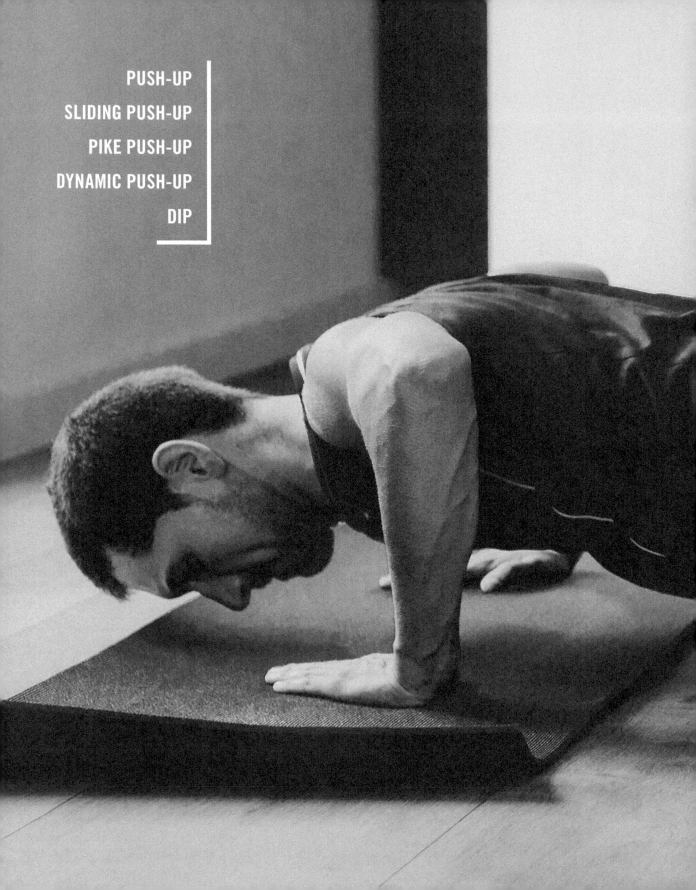

The multijoint movements in this chapter's exercises will build your pec-torals, deltoids, triceps, and other stabilizing muscles in your upper body. There are two main types of pushes: horizontal and vertical. A good workout program uses a balanced mix of both, which is why I've included exercises like dips, shoulder presses, and many variations on the push-up. In order to

PUSH

have a strong push, you have to have a stable platform to push from. Think about playing chicken in a pool on your friend's shoulders. If the person on the bottom isn't stable, the person on top won't be able to push with any leverage. Your core is like the person on the bottom, so you have to make it strong before you can ask the person on top—your upper body—to perform well. If you're having trouble with any of these exercises, make sure you've adequately trained your core before you start blaming any push muscles.

PUSH-UP

Primary muscle groups: Pectorals, Deltoids
Secondary muscle groups: Triceps, Abdominals

46
BASE

ELEVATED PUSH-UP

47
INTERMEDIATE

CLASSIC PUSH-UP

48
ADVANCED

PUSH-UP WITH SHOULDER TAP

These variations of the push-up challenge your chest, shoulders, and triceps to provide the power for your motion, while your core provides the stabilization your arms need to push. Here you'll start with an elevated, regressed version of the push-up to perfect your form before moving on to the classic push-up and then a harder version with a stability challenge. All of these variations are classified as horizontal pushes.

46 / ELEVATED PUSH-UP

Many people don't think of a push-up as an advanced exercise, but it's harder than you might think to do one correctly. With all the stabilization it requires, a push-up isn't really a basic exercise—it's actually a progression of the gym's traditional horizontal push, the bench press. If you don't have the stability or strength to perform several repetitions, you can start off by pushing up from an elevated position using a bench or counter. That way, your core still gets the practice of hip and spine stabilization, but your chest and shoulders don't have to work as hard to lift your body. Once your core is strong enough to keep your spine and pelvis neutral consistently, you can move up to the classic push-up (47).

GOAL: You want to be able to do at least 20 repetitions *and* hold a plank position (01) for at least 1 minute before progressing to the Classic Push-Up (47).

1 Place your hands on a solid elevated structure like a bench or counter. To find the correct position for your feet, bend your arms to replicate the "down" part of a push-up and then place your feet so that the edge of the counter lies just below your sternum.

2 With your pelvis in a neutral position, press through your arms, fully extending your elbows. **A**

3 When you're ready, slowly lower your body in a controlled manner toward the counter.

4 As your chest comes within a few inches of the counter, press through your arms and fully extend your elbows again. **B**

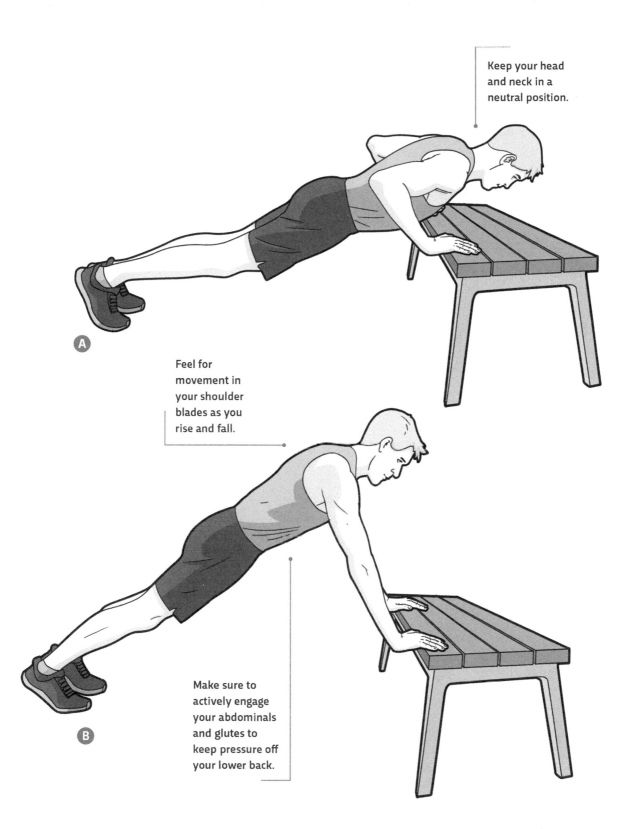

Keep your head and neck in a neutral position.

A

Feel for movement in your shoulder blades as you rise and fall.

Make sure to actively engage your abdominals and glutes to keep pressure off your lower back.

B

47 / CLASSIC PUSH-UP

This exercise is a staple of calisthenics. You'll go on to use many variations of it, so it's important to master this more basic version. It uses the chest, shoulders, and triceps to press the full weight of your body while forcing your core to stabilize you throughout the entire motion. Remember that without a stable core, these muscles have nothing to push against, and the level of strength you can achieve diminishes greatly.

GOAL: **When you can do 20 repetitions with perfect form, you're ready to try the Push-Up with Shoulder Tap (48).**

1 Start in a plank position facing the floor with your arms straight out in front of you, your knees locked, and your feet together on the floor. **A**

----

2 Keeping your pelvis in a neutral position, use your arms to lower your shoulders and hips as one unit toward the floor.

----

3 When your chest is about 3 inches from the floor, press through your palms, continuing to move your shoulders and hips as one unit, and return to the starting position. **B**

Keep your head
and neck in a
neutral position.

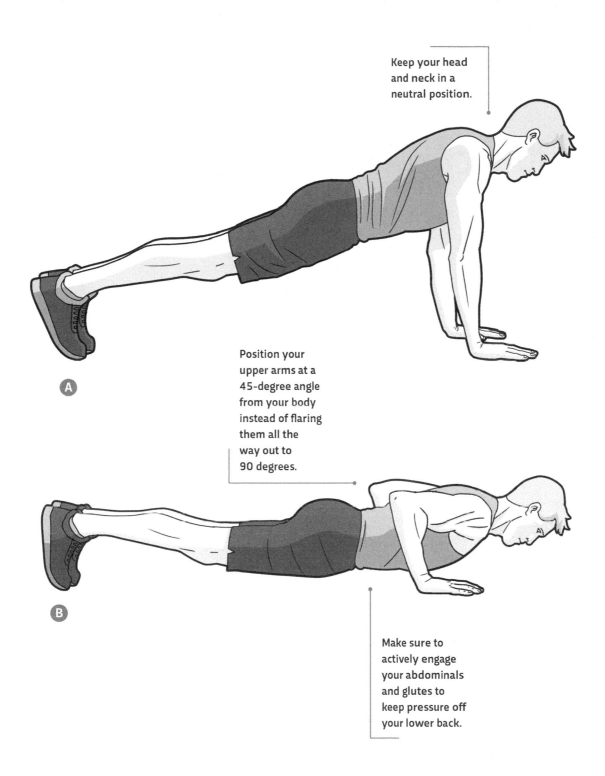

A

Position your
upper arms at a
45-degree angle
from your body
instead of flaring
them all the
way out to
90 degrees.

B

Make sure to
actively engage
your abdominals
and glutes to
keep pressure off
your lower back.

48 / PUSH-UP WITH SHOULDER TAP

This variation on the classic push-up (47) adds a stability challenge by decreasing your base of support. Between each push, you slowly lift one arm from the ground and tap the opposite shoulder. You'll probably have to spread your feet wide at first to regain some of the stability you'll lose by lifting one arm. But as you build your strength, you can slowly narrow the spread of your feet, increasing the difficulty of the exercise and working your core harder.

GOAL: Work toward getting your feet 12 inches apart or closer. Aim to do 10 taps on each side.

1 Start in a plank position facing the floor with your arms straight out in front of you, your knees locked, and your feet at shoulder-width or wider on the floor.

2 Keeping your pelvis in a neutral position, use your arms to lower your shoulders and hips as one unit toward the floor.

3 When your chest is about 3 inches from the floor, press through your palms, continuing to move your shoulders and hips as one unit, and return to the starting position.

4 Before starting the next repetition, lift one hand and tap the opposite shoulder. **A** Switch your tapping hand at the end of each repetition.

For an extra challenge, try tapping both shoulders before doing the next push-up.

Make sure your hips don't rotate to accommodate for the loss of your hand as a contact point with the ground.

As you get better, slowly narrow your feet to increase the difficulty. Elevating your feet also makes this exercise harder.

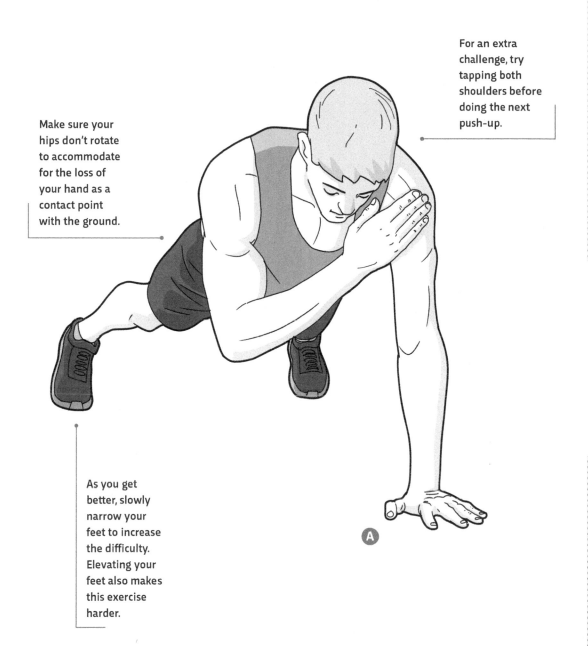

A

SLIDING PUSH-UP

Primary muscle groups: Pectorals, Deltoids
Secondary muscle groups: Triceps, Abdominals

49
BASE

HORIZONTAL SLIDING PUSH-UP FROM KNEES

50
INTERMEDIATE

HORIZONTAL SLIDING PUSH-UP FROM FEET

51
INTERMEDIATE

VERTICAL SLIDING PUSH-UP

Sliding push-ups are a modification of the classic push-up. These horizontal push exercises work the shoulders in a fly-like motion. You do them on a mat with a towel under one hand so that you can slide that hand back and forth. Here you'll start with a regression done from the knees so you can get used to the movement and perfect your form. You'll do the next level from your feet, then switch to a vertical slide for some directional variation.

49 / HORIZONTAL SLIDING PUSH-UP FROM KNEES

As its name implies, this push-up is done from the knees, which decreases the challenge on the stability of your core and shoulders while you build strength in your chest and arms. You use the same basic motion as a push-up (47), but you keep a towel (or washcloth, napkin, etc.) under each hand, and when you drop into a push-up, slide one hand out to the side, reaching as far as you can while keeping your sliding arm straight. As you return to the starting position, you try to keep the sliding arm straight, which forces the chest and shoulders to work from a different angle, maximizing the exercise's benefits.

GOAL: Aim to do 10 repetitions on each side before progressing from your knees to your feet (50).

1 On a mat, assume a modified push-up position with your knees on the ground and your hands lined up slightly wider than your shoulders. Put a towel under each hand. **A**

2 Slowly drop into a push-up, and at the same time, slide one hand laterally until your chest is a few inches from the floor. **B**

3 Press through both palms as you squeeze with the chest and return your hand to its starting position. **A** Make sure to keep the sliding arm straight, forcing a different muscle contraction from the stable arm.

4 Switch to the other side and repeat, alternating hands on each repetition.

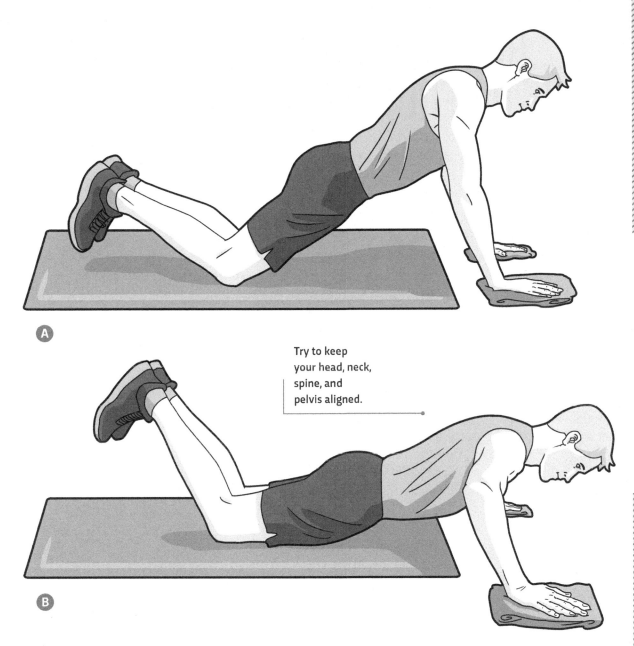

A

Try to keep
your head, neck,
spine, and
pelvis aligned.

B

50 / HORIZONTAL SLIDING PUSH-UP FROM FEET

In this variation, you do the sliding push-up from your feet instead of your knees. Now that gravity has more leverage to pull you down, you'll feel the intense amount of core stabilization and chest strength needed to perform the press. With this kind of stress running through your shoulders, it's imperative that you keep your arms rotated outward, meaning the insides of your elbows are pointing out in front of you rather than in toward each other. Rotating them inward increases the risk of a shoulder impingement or rotator cuff injury. To encourage outward rotation, make sure that when you bend your arms, they fall close to your body rather than flaring way out to the side.

GOAL: Aim to do 10 repetitions on each side.

1 On a hard surface, assume a plank position with your hands lined up under your shoulders, your knees locked, and your feet on the ground. Keep a towel under each hand. **A**

----

2 Slowly drop into a push-up, and at the same time, slide one hand out laterally until your chest is a few inches from the floor. **B**

----

3 Press through your palms as you squeeze with your chest and slide your hand back to its starting position.

----

4 Switch to the other side and repeat, alternating hands on each repetition.

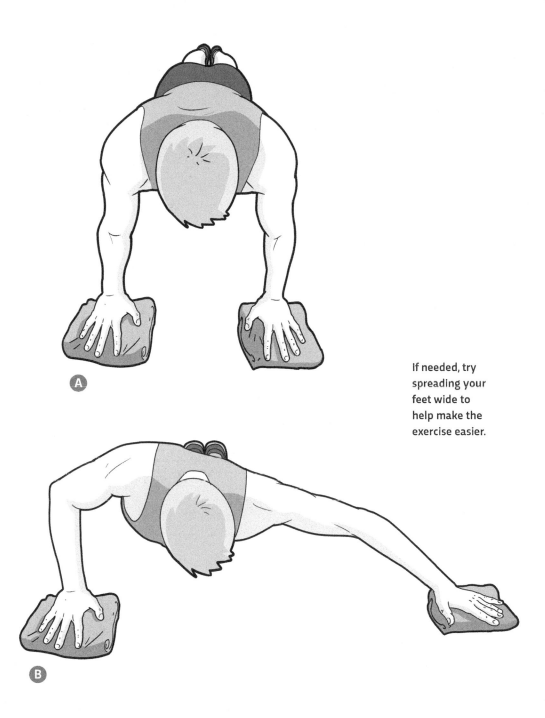

A

B

If needed, try spreading your feet wide to help make the exercise easier.

51 / VERTICAL SLIDING PUSH-UP

This variation is similar to the previous one (50), but your hand will slide up overhead instead of out to the side. You may need to do this sliding push-up with a slightly wider foot base because the vertical slide doesn't give you as much stability as the horizontal one, but that lack of stability is also what makes this move so great for building core strength. The vertical slide takes away your chest's leverage, forcing your lats to support the movement.

GOAL: 10 repetitions on each side

1 On a hard surface, assume a plank position with your hands lined up under your shoulders, your knees locked, and your feet on the ground. Keep a towel under each hand. **A**

2 Slowly drop into a push-up, and at the same time, slide one hand out vertically overhead until your chest is a few inches from the floor. **B**

3 Press through the palm as you squeeze with your chest and armpit to return the sliding hand to its starting position. **A**

4 Switch to the other side and repeat, alternating hands on each repetition.

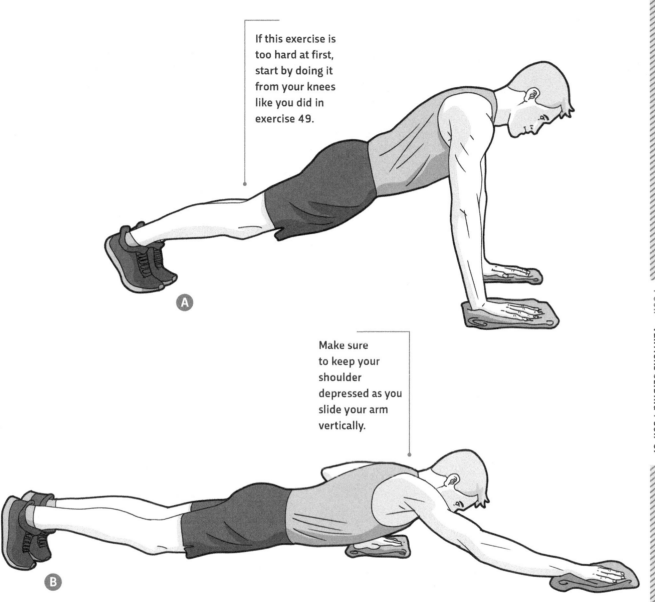

If this exercise is too hard at first, start by doing it from your knees like you did in exercise 49.

A

Make sure to keep your shoulder depressed as you slide your arm vertically.

B

PIKE PUSH-UP

Primary muscle groups: Deltoids, Pectorals
Secondary muscle group: Triceps

52
BASE

BENT KNEE PIKE PUSH-UP

53
INTERMEDIATE

STRAIGHT LEG PIKE PUSH-UP

54
ADVANCED

HANDSTAND PUSH-UP

Doing something in a "pike position" means you're bending at the waist but keeping your legs straight. This version of the push-up is classified as a vertical push, and it targets your shoulders. Pike push-ups build up to handstand push-ups (54), but they also allow you to do many more repetitions and give you a slightly larger range of motion than true handstand push-ups do, so I actually prefer the first two exercises to the final variation here. You can do these from the ground or on a step for varying degrees of difficulty.

52 / BENT KNEE PIKE PUSH-UP

You do this variation from a step with your knees bent to limit the amount of body weight you put over your arms and shoulders. When you're doing any pressing with your arms, it's important to remember to keep your shoulders pulled down toward your hips and not let them get up around your ears. The same rules apply when you're upside down in an exercise like this one.

GOAL: When you can do 20 repetitions comfortably, you're ready to attempt it with straight legs (53).

1 Stand with your back to a bench or other elevated surface. Bend forward, place your hands on the ground, and place your feet on top of the elevated surface, bending your hips and knees to align your body over the hands and shoulders. **A**

----

2 While keeping your arms rotated outward with the insides of your elbows facing out away from your feet, bend your elbows and lower your head toward the ground. **B**

----

3 Just before the top of your head touches the ground, press through your palms and return to the starting position. **A**

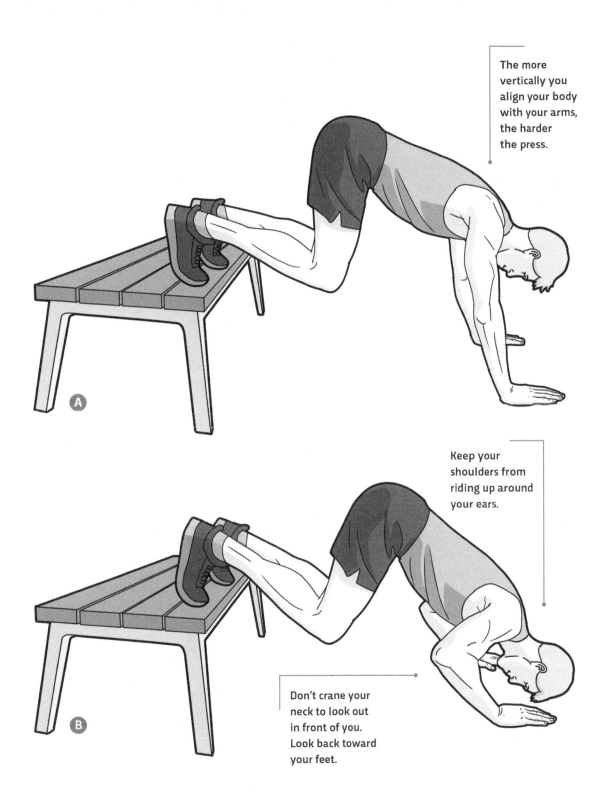

The more vertically you align your body with your arms, the harder the press.

Keep your shoulders from riding up around your ears.

Don't crane your neck to look out in front of you. Look back toward your feet.

53 / STRAIGHT LEG PIKE PUSH-UP

You can do this variation from a step or from the ground, depending on your hip mobility. You want to have a neutral spine, so if your lower back has to round excessively when your feet are on the ground, elevate them onto a step. The straighter you can stack your spine on top of your arms and shoulders, the more difficult the push-up—and the closer you are to doing a handstand push-up (54). Again, keep your shoulders pulled down toward your hips and not up around your ears when doing any pressing, even when you're upside down. And keep your arms rotated outward by not letting your elbows flare too wide.

GOAL: Get very comfortable with doing 20 repetitions and supporting your weight with your shoulders before you attempt the Handstand Push-Up (54).

1 Place your hands on the ground, and move your feet up as close to your hands as you can while still keeping your knees straight and your spine from rounding. Ⓐ Your body should form a sort of upside-down V. If you need to, put your feet on top of a step or other elevated surface.

2 Keeping your legs locked, shift as much weight as you can over your hands and shoulders.

3 Bend your elbows and lower your head toward the ground while rotating your arms outward by turning the insides of your elbows toward your face and away from your feet. Ⓑ

4 Just before the top of your head touches the ground, press through your palms and return to the starting position. Ⓐ

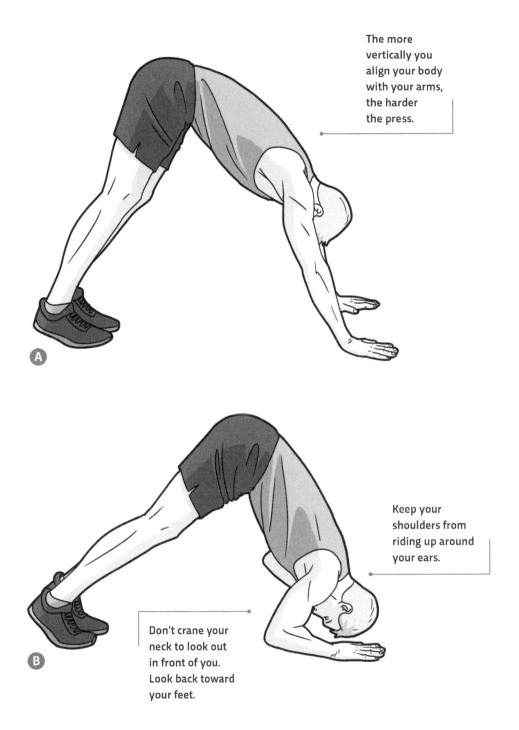

The more vertically you align your body with your arms, the harder the press.

A

Keep your shoulders from riding up around your ears.

Don't crane your neck to look out in front of you. Look back toward your feet.

B

54 / HANDSTAND PUSH-UP

This variation is about as vertical a push as anyone can do and is possibly the most difficult exercise you'll encounter in any typical bodyweight training program. Unless you're a gymnast and can comfortably do a handstand, you'll need to do this in front of a wall to keep your balance. Please use caution when attempting this. Falling on your head can result in serious injury.

GOAL: 10 repetitions

1 Stand facing a wall, and place your hands on the floor 12 to 18 inches in front of it.

2 Fling your legs up so that the wall is supporting you in a full handstand. **A**

3 Bend your elbows and lower your head toward the ground while rotating your arms outward by turning the insides of your elbows toward your face. **B**

4 Just before the top of your head touches the ground, **C** press through your palms and return to the starting standing position.

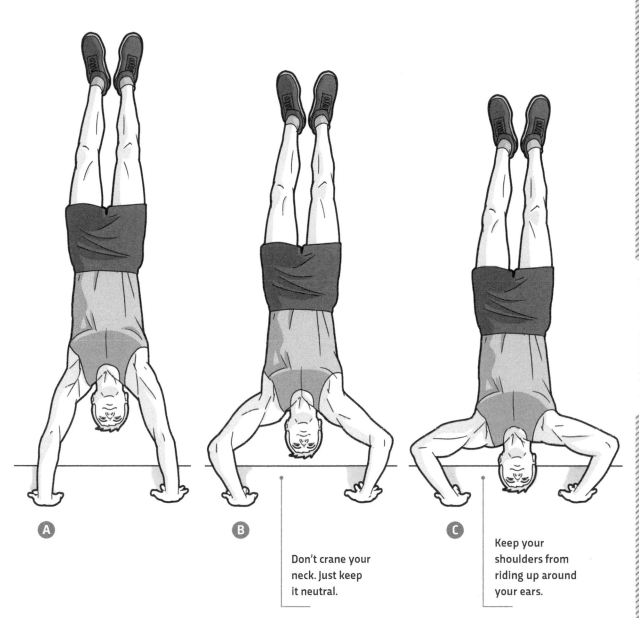

A

B

Don't crane your neck. Just keep it neutral.

C

Keep your shoulders from riding up around your ears.

DYNAMIC PUSH-UP

Primary muscle groups: Pectorals, Deltoids
Secondary muscle groups: Triceps, Abdominals

55
BASE

**T
PUSH-UP**

56
INTERMEDIATE

**SIDE TO SIDE
PUSH-UP**

57
ADVANCED

**SCOOPING
PUSH-UP**

Dynamic, or moving, push-ups are another variation on the push-up. They have the added challenge of stabilizing the body as it moves through a weight shift during the push-up. Two of the variations have a horizontal shifting pattern, while the third moves through a fluid range of vertical motion, challenging your shoulders' strength and stability.

55 / T PUSH-UP

This variation combines the work of a classic push-up (47) with a side plank (02). Between each push up, the shoulders and core must stabilize the body through a horizontal weight shift into a full side plank from the hands.

GOAL: Work toward doing 10 repetitions on each side.

1 Position yourself in a basic push-up position, but with feet about 12 inches apart. Perform a classic push-up, **A** and as you finish the press, **B** lift one hand, rotate through your hips, land on the sides of your feet, and come to rest in a side plank position. **C**

2 Hold for one second, then rotate back to the classic push-up position. **B**

3 Perform another push-up, **A** but this time as you finish the press, rotate in the opposite direction and come to rest in a side plank on the other side.

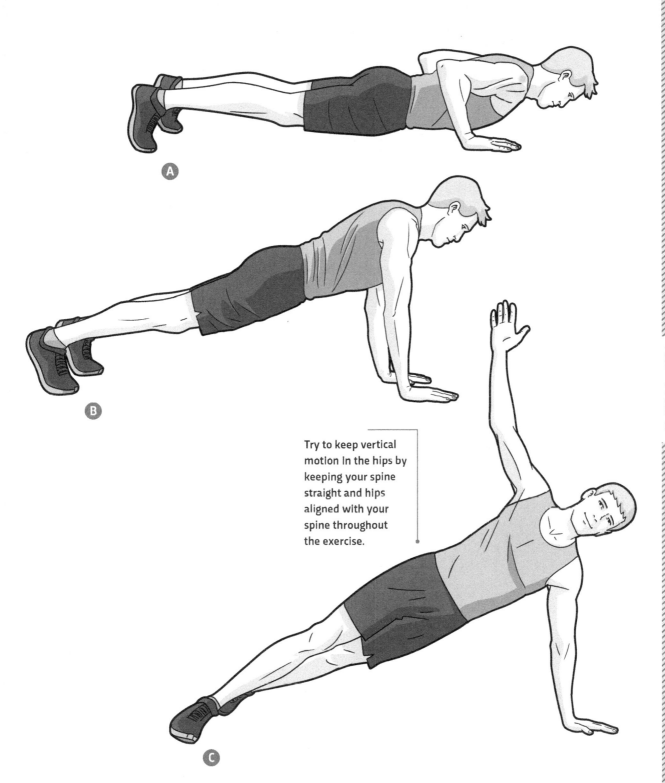

A

B

Try to keep vertical motion in the hips by keeping your spine straight and hips aligned with your spine throughout the exercise.

C

56 / SIDE TO SIDE PUSH-UP

This is a fun variation that again challenges your body with a horizontal shift. You perform it like a classic push-up (47), except that as you lower yourself, you shift your body to one side and position one shoulder directly over the hand so that the bottom of the push-up is over to one side. Start with a wider foot base, bringing the feet closer together as you progress.

GOAL: Gradually decrease your foot base until you can do the exercise with your feet together. Work toward doing 10 repetitions on each side.

1 Start in a push-up position with your feet 12 inches apart. **A** As you lower yourself into the push-up, smoothly shift your body laterally so you land at the bottom with your right shoulder positioned directly over your right hand. **B**

2 As you press back up to the starting position, smoothly shift back to center so that you finish the press at the same time you finish the shift. Alternate and repeat on the left side. **C**

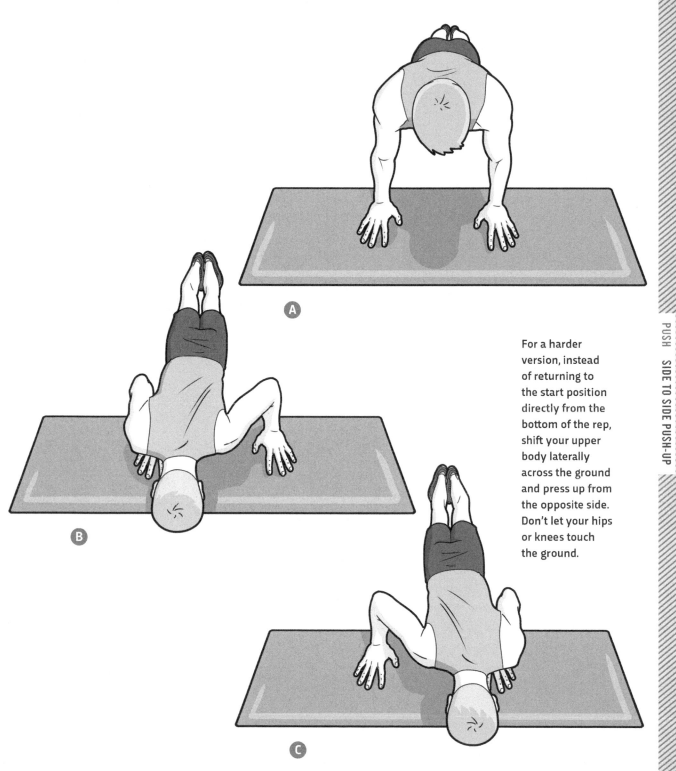

A

B

For a harder version, instead of returning to the start position directly from the bottom of the rep, shift your upper body laterally across the ground and press up from the opposite side. Don't let your hips or knees touch the ground.

C

191

57 / SCOOPING PUSH-UP

Unlike the first two variations, the scooping push-up offers a dynamic vertical motion for the chest and shoulders to control. It starts in a downward dog position rather than a plank and forces you to lower yourself while shifting your bodyweight forward. As your chest passes your hands, you press your arms back out, extending your spine into a modified cobra position in the scooping motion that gives this variation its name. Then you just shift your hips upward, slide your shoulders back behind your hands, and lower your head, and you're ready to start over again. If you feel pain or pressure in your lower back or shoulders, this may not be the best variation for you just yet.

GOAL: 20 repetitions

1 Start on your hands and knees, then straighten your legs and press your hips upward so you form a sort of upside-down V (downward dog). **A** Find a straight line from your hands through your arms, shoulders, and spine all the way to your hips.

- -

2 With your arms rotated outward so that the insides of your elbows are toward your face, bend your elbows (they should point down toward your feet) and bring your shoulders toward your hands. **B**

- -

3 As you pass your hands, **C** perform a scooping motion by pressing through your arms and lifting only your head and shoulders, **D** leaving your hips just a few inches from the ground. Take a moment to stretch with your spine in extension. **E**

- -

4 Press your hips back upward and lower your shoulders until you're back in your starting position. **A**

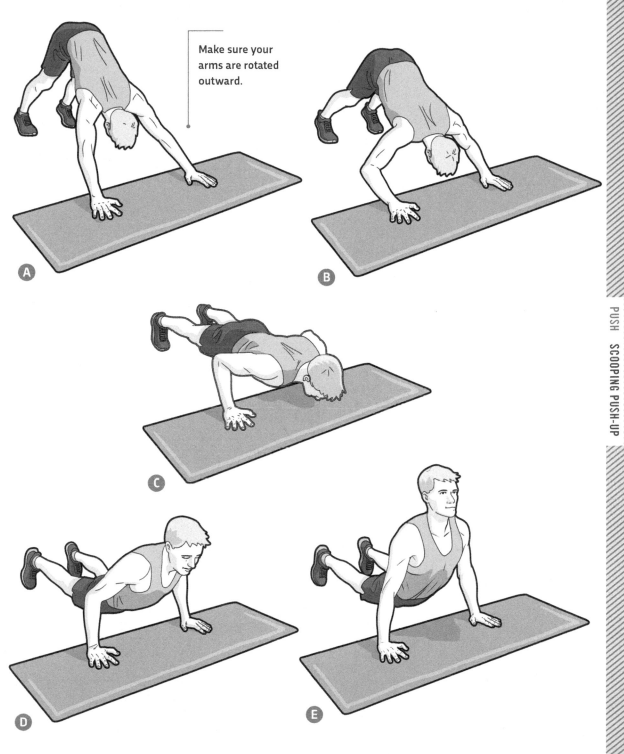

Make sure your arms are rotated outward.

A

B

C

D

E

DIP

Primary muscle groups: Deltoids, Triceps
Secondary muscle group: Pectorals

58
BASE

**BENT KNEE
BENCH DIP**

59
INTERMEDIATE

**STRAIGHT LEG
BENCH DIP**

60
ADVANCED

**PARALLEL
BAR DIP**

The dip is another vertical push, and it's a great way to work your triceps and deltoids. Dips can be tough on the shoulder joint, however, so if you have improper mobility or poor upper-body posture, proceed with caution. If they cause you pain, stick to the pike push-ups. However, if you do have the mobility and alignment to do dips well, you can do them in many ways, including from a bench, step, or parallel bars. Here you'll do two variations that use a bench and finish by supporting your full body weight on the parallel bars.

58 / BENT KNEE BENCH DIP

These dips are a good place to begin because you do them with your knees bent and your feet flat, so if your upper body isn't strong enough to hold most of your body weight, you can easily support yourself with your legs. You'll need a bench, step, or retaining wall of at least knee height to do this variation. Keep the physiological limitations of your shoulders in mind during these dips. When a joint like the elbow extends to the limit of its range of motion, it's stopped by bone, but when you reach the end of your shoulder's range of motion, there's only soft tissue. You don't want to stress it too hard, or you could end up with an injury.

GOAL: When you can do 20 repetitions without any assistance from your legs, you're ready for the Straight Leg Bench Dip (59).

1 With your back to a bench, step, or retaining wall of at least knee height, squat down and place the heels of your palms on the top surface with your fingers coming down over the edge. **A**

2 Slowly walk your feet out until you can use your arms to comfortably lower your body while maintaining a vertical spine without scraping up against the edge of the structure.

3 Keeping your knees bent and your feet flat on the ground, use the movement of your elbows and shoulders to lower your body. **B** Don't let your upper arm go past the point where it's parallel with the ground.

4 Keeping your chest up and your shoulders down, press through your hands, straightening your arms and lifting your body back to its starting position. **A**

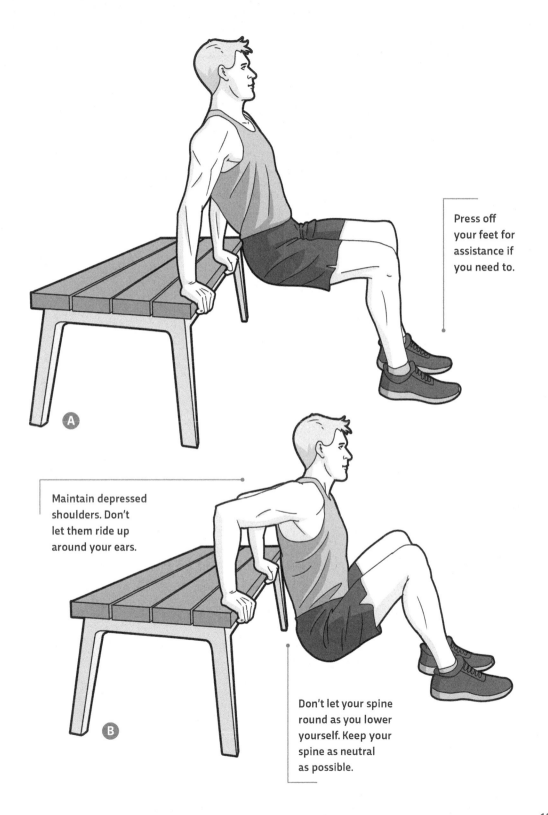

Press off your feet for assistance if you need to.

Maintain depressed shoulders. Don't let them ride up around your ears.

Don't let your spine round as you lower yourself. Keep your spine as neutral as possible.

59 / STRAIGHT LEG BENCH DIP

This variation is also done off a bench or step, but this time you keep your legs straight so that only the heels of your feet are on the ground. This position keeps your legs from helping you and forces your upper body to provide all the strength necessary to complete the movement. The optimal position for your legs is one that lets your spine remain mostly vertical through the motion as it passes very close to the ledge you have your hands on.

GOAL: 20 repetitions

1 With your back to a bench, step, or retaining wall of at least knee height, squat down and place the heels of your palms on the top surface with your fingers coming down over the edge.

----

2 Slowly walk your feet out. Straighten your legs, and place your heels on the ground at a distance that lets you use your arms to comfortably lower your body while maintaining a vertical spine without scraping up against the edge of your structure. **A**

----

3 Use the movement of your elbows and shoulders to lower your body, keeping your spine as neutral and vertical as possible. **B** Don't let your upper arm go past the point where it's parallel with the ground.

----

4 Keeping your chest up and your shoulders down, press through your hands, straightening your arms and lifting your body back to its starting position. **A**

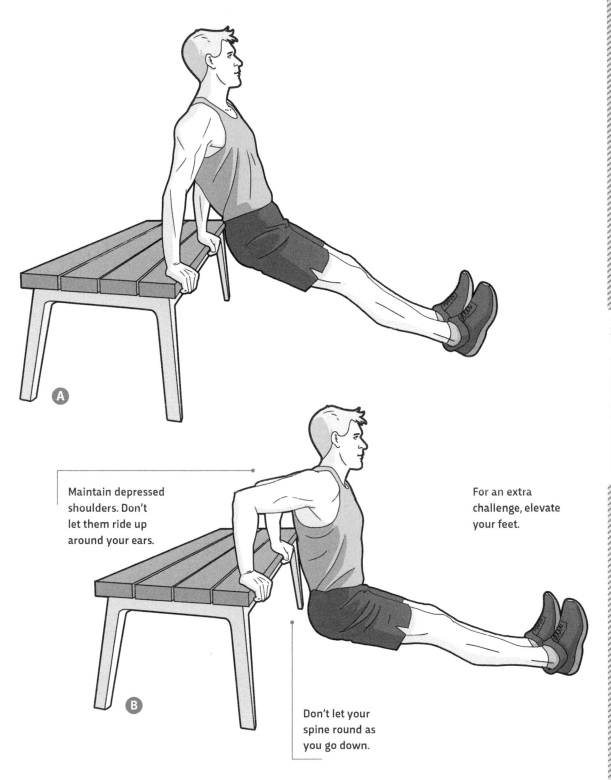

Maintain depressed shoulders. Don't let them ride up around your ears.

For an extra challenge, elevate your feet.

Don't let your spine round as you go down.

60 / PARALLEL BAR DIP

These dips require the use of parallel bars and force you to press your entire body weight. By leaning your body forward, you recruit more chest muscles into the movement, and by leaning back, you use more triceps and deltoids. Again, be careful as you descend toward your maximum depth, because the soft tissue of the shoulder capsule doesn't have much protection from hyperextension. If you feel pain, you can decrease your depth or omit the exercise altogether.

GOAL: Build up to doing 20 repetitions.

1 Stand between parallel bars with one hand on each bar. Straighten your arms and lift your body into a tall position. A

- -

2 While supporting your entire body weight, bend your elbows and shoulders to slowly lower your body. B Do not lower yourself past the point where your upper arm is parallel with the ground.

- -

3 Keeping your chest up and your shoulders down, press through your hands, straightening your arms and lifting your body back to its starting position. A

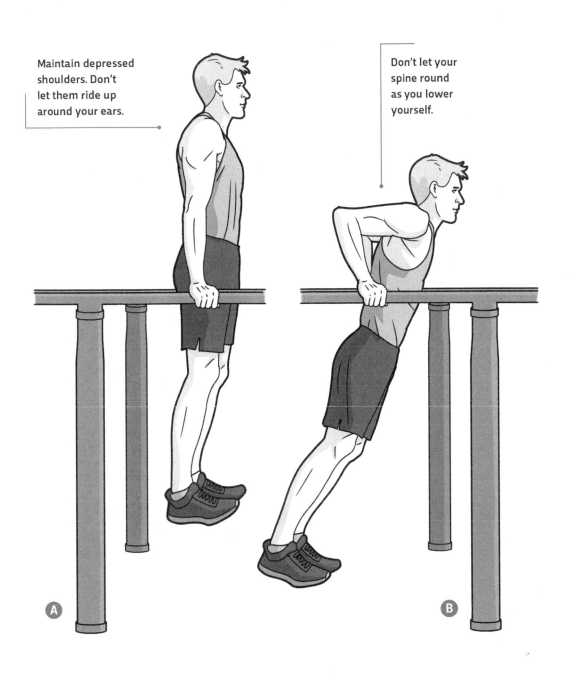

Maintain depressed shoulders. Don't let them ride up around your ears.

Don't let your spine round as you lower yourself.

Ⓐ

Ⓑ

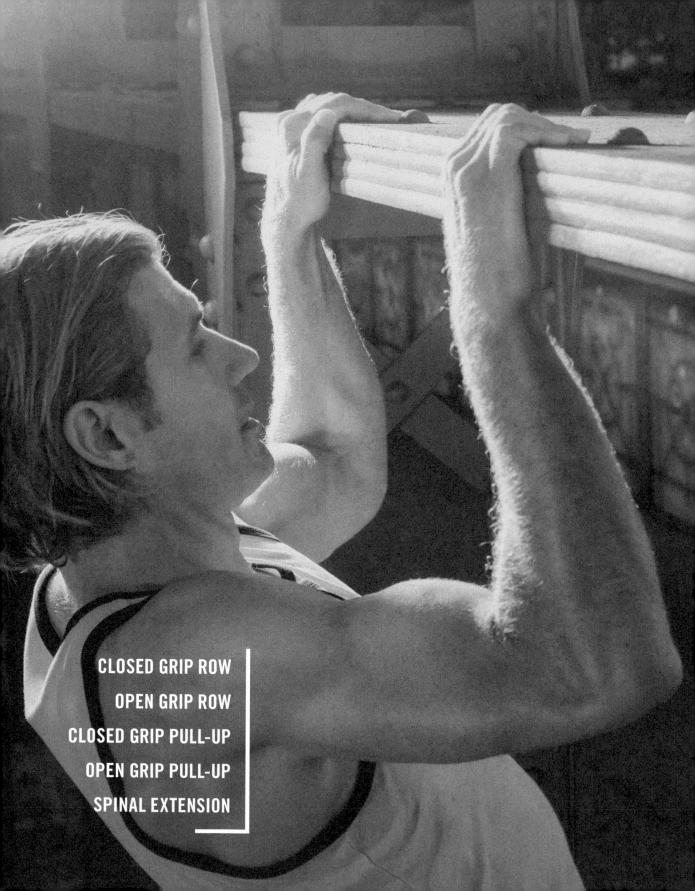

CLOSED GRIP ROW
OPEN GRIP ROW
CLOSED GRIP PULL-UP
OPEN GRIP PULL-UP
SPINAL EXTENSION

SEVEN

Just like each action has an equal and opposite reaction, every push has its pull, and any solid training program must balance the two. Unfortunately, it's not as easy to do pulling exercises at home, so some of these will require you to go outside and get creative. A pull-up bar is a great resource, but you'll also want something about half that height that you can hang from to perform

PULL

more of a horizontal pull, known as a *row*. These exercises target your back, shoulders, and arms. Many of them require you to "pack your shoulders," meaning you pull your shoulder blades back a bit until you find a stable—but not immobile—feeling within the ball-and-socket joint of your shoulder. This prevents injury and reinforces good form by keeping your shoulder blades from protracting too far, which would cause your shoulders to elevate and your arms to rotate inward. And, as always, a weak core will greatly reduce the amount of strength you can pull with, so make sure you have your core under control before you start on the more advanced pulling exercises.

CLOSED GRIP ROW

Primary muscle groups: Trapezius, Deltoids
Secondary muscle group: Biceps

61

BASE

**BENT KNEE
CLOSED GRIP
ROW**

62

INTERMEDIATE

**STRAIGHT LEG
CLOSED GRIP
ROW**

63

ADVANCED

**SWITCH
GRIP
ROW**

These versions of the row use a grip called the closed, supinated, or reverse grip, putting your arms naturally into an outwardly rotated position, which is much safer for your shoulders. They also challenge your biceps a little more. You can do these rows from varying bar heights as well as with straight or bent legs to control difficulty. The lower the bar and the straighter your legs, the more difficult the movement.

61 / BENT KNEE CLOSED GRIP ROW

This variation is a great option if the only bar you have to row from is low. As the height of the bar lowers, the row exercise becomes exponentially more difficult, and bending your knees is a great way to make things easier. Grabbing the bar with a closed (palms-up) grip will help you strengthen the external rotators of your arm, because they have to stabilize you while you move through the full range of motion. You'll feel your biceps working harder, as they now have a longer stretch and thus become more active.

GOAL: 20 repetitions

1 Grip your chosen bar with your palms up, and hang underneath it. Bend your knees so your legs roughly form a 90-degree angle. Align your body so there's a straight line through your knees, hips, shoulders, and head. **A**

----

2 Engage your trapezius muscles by pulling your shoulders down toward your hips, slightly retracting your shoulder blade to find stability in your shoulder.

----

3 Pull your chest toward the bar **B** by bending your arms and pulling back your shoulder blades, being careful not to elevate your shoulders.

----

4 Once the bar touches your lower chest, slowly lower your body back to the starting position, being careful not to extend your shoulders too far. **A**

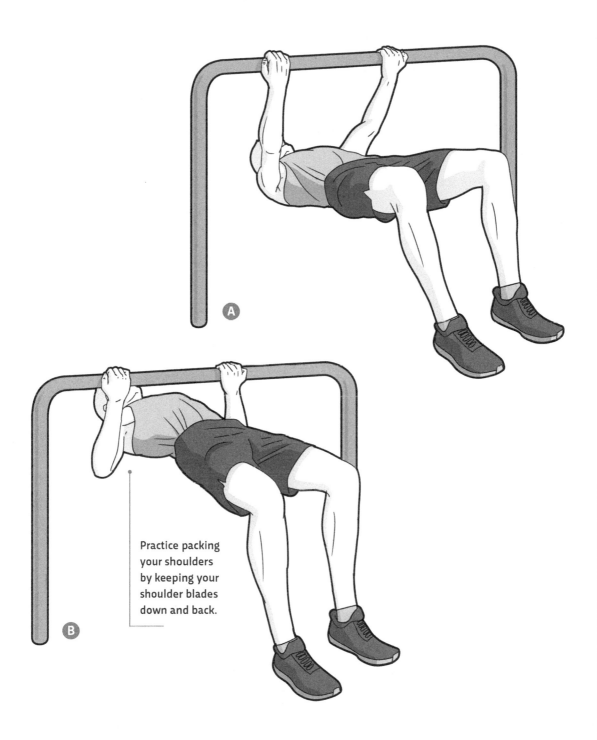

Practice packing
your shoulders
by keeping your
shoulder blades
down and back.

62 / STRAIGHT LEG CLOSED GRIP ROW

In this variation, you use the palms-up grip and keep your body straight under the bar as you row. The bar should make contact with or come close to the lower portion of your chest. If it's at your upper chest or collarbone, you're misaligned or elevating your shoulders too much during the row. You keep your legs out straight and use your heels as the pivot point of the movement. This variation requires much more core stability than the previous exercise. Be careful not to lead the row with your hips. Instead, keep your hips down and lead with your shoulders, keeping your body in an upside-down plank position.

GOAL: 20 repetitions

1 Grip your chosen bar with your palms up, and hang underneath it. Straighten your legs, dig your heels into the ground, and flex your feet up toward your face. Align your body so there's a straight line all the way through your ankles, knees, hips, shoulders, and head. (A)

2 Engage your trapezius muscles by pulling your shoulders down toward your hips, slightly retracting your shoulder blade to find stability in your shoulder.

3 Pull your chest toward the bar by bending your arms and pulling back your shoulder blades, being careful not to elevate your shoulders. (B)

4 Once the bar touches your lower chest, slowly lower your body back to the starting position, being careful not to extend your shoulders too far. (A)

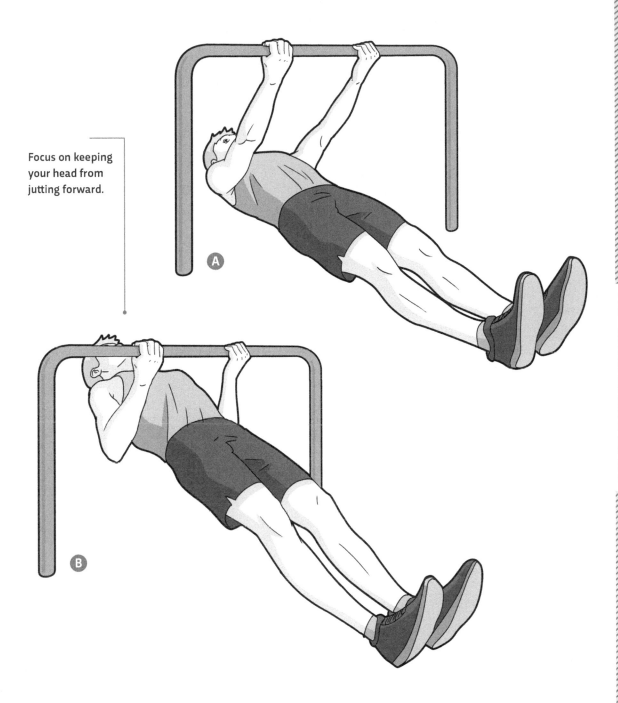

Focus on keeping your head from jutting forward.

A

B

63 / SWITCH GRIP ROW

This variation is a great way to add a little difficulty if the bar you're working with feels too high, but it can get a little risky, so proceed with caution. For the switch grip row, you have to pull yourself up with enough speed that you generate the momentum necessary to let go of the bar at the top of the motion and quickly switch your grip for every rep.

GOAL: Work toward doing 20 repetitions.

1 Grip your chosen bar with your palms facing away from you (closed grip), straighten your legs, dig your heels into the ground, and flex your feet up toward your face. Align your body so there's a straight line all the way through your ankles, knees, hips, shoulders, and head. **A**

2 Engage your trapezius muscles by pulling your shoulders down toward your hips, slightly retracting your shoulder blade to find stability in your shoulder.

3 Pull your chest toward the bar at fairly high speed **B** so that as you reach the top of your motion, you can quickly let go with both hands and grab the bar with your palms facing away from you (open grip). **C**

4 Catch yourself with the new grip, and absorb your weight as you transition smoothly back to the starting position. **D**

5 Repeat, this time switching your grip from palms up to palms down. A rep with each grip counts as one.

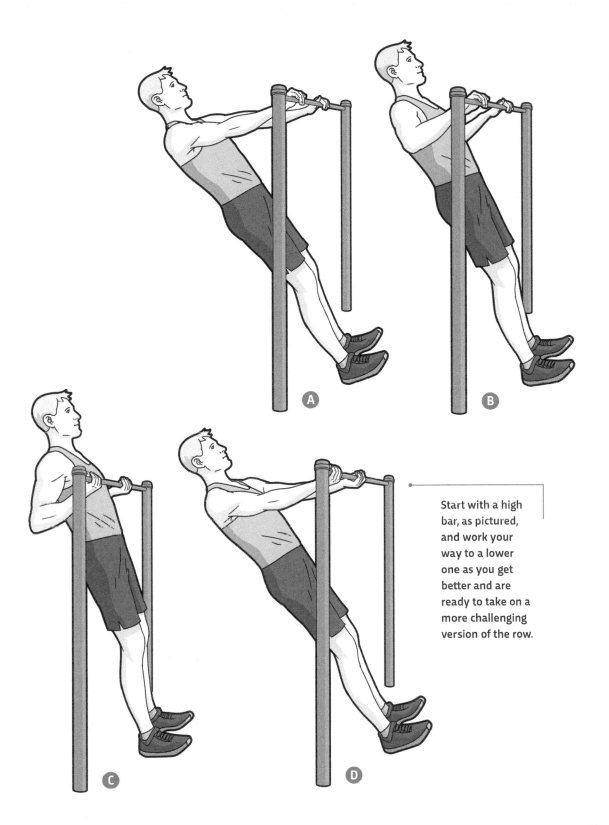

Start with a high bar, as pictured, and work your way to a lower one as you get better and are ready to take on a more challenging version of the row.

OPEN GRIP ROW

Primary muscle groups: Trapezius, Deltoids
Secondary muscle group: Biceps

64
BASE

BENT KNEE OPEN GRIP ROW

65
INTERMEDIATE

STRAIGHT LEG OPEN GRIP ROW

66
ADVANCED

ONE ARM OPEN GRIP ROW

This is a traditional row with a pronated (palms-down) grip. It's important to have good awareness of your spine and neck position when building a good rowing pattern. Make sure not to jut your head forward through any of the motions. You should also try to keep your hips neutral by firing your glutes and abs together just like you would in a plank (01). You'll move quickly through these variations as you get better at them. You'll start with a bent-knee variation to reduce the amount of weight you have to row, then move on to a straight-leg version before finally tackling a one-arm row.

64 / BENT KNEE OPEN GRIP ROW

This variation lets you bend your legs to reduce the amount of weight you need to pull. You'll need a sturdy bar to work from, about 4-feet high, give or take a few inches depending on your height and arm length. As you finish your row, the bar should land at lower-chest level. If it lands at midchest level or up near your collarbone, your shoulder blades are forced up around your ears, which will prevent you from reaching your true strength potential. Like you do during a push-up, always try to keep your shoulder blades pulled down toward your hips.

GOAL: 20 repetitions

1 Grip your chosen bar with your palms facing away from you, and hang underneath it. Bend your knees so your legs form roughly a 90-degree angle. Align your body so there's a straight line between your knees, hips, shoulders, and head. **A**

2 Engage your trapezius muscles by pulling your shoulders down toward your hips, slightly retracting your shoulder blades to find stability in your shoulders.

3 Pull your chest toward the bar by bending your arms and pulling back your shoulder blades, being careful not to elevate your shoulders. **B**

4 Once the bar touches your lower chest, slowly lower your body to its starting position, **A** being careful not to extend your shoulders too far.

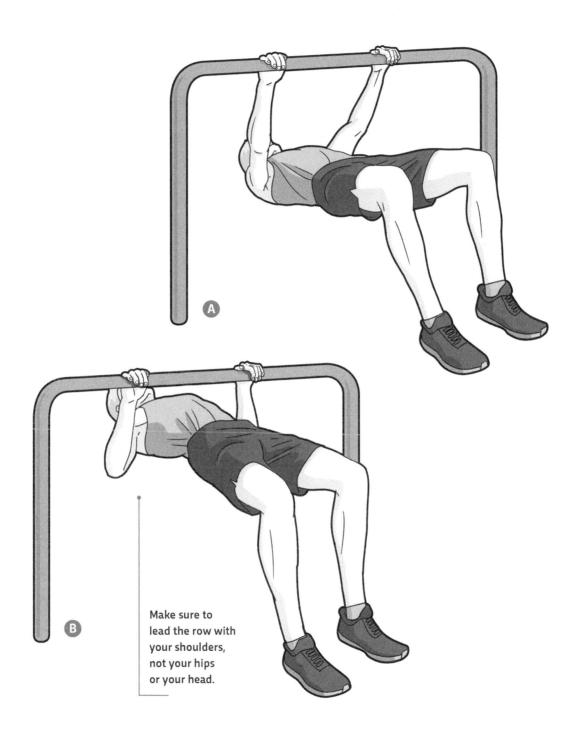

Make sure to lead the row with your shoulders, not your hips or your head.

65 / STRAIGHT LEG OPEN GRIP ROW

In this variation, you'll squeeze your legs straight and row yourself in an upside-down plank position. You'll have to pull an amount much closer to your full body weight than you did in the bent knee row (64). You may have to walk your feet out a little farther, but the bar should still come to your lower chest as you finish the row. Remember to practice supporting your arms from your back muscles, and don't let your shoulder blades protract too far.

GOAL: You should be comfortable with doing at least 20 repetitions before you attempt the One Arm Open Grip Row (66).

1 Grip your chosen bar with your palms facing away from you, and hang underneath it. Straighten your legs, dig your heels into the ground, and flex your feet so that your toes point up toward your face. **A** Align your body so there's a straight line between your ankles, knees, hips, shoulders, and head.

----

2 Engage your trapezius muscles by pulling your shoulders down toward your hips, slightly retracting your shoulder blades to find stability in your shoulders.

----

3 Pull your chest toward the bar by bending your arms and pulling back your shoulder blades, **B** being careful not to elevate your shoulders or push your head forward.

----

4 Once the bar touches your lower chest, slowly return to the starting position, **A** being careful not to extend your shoulders too far.

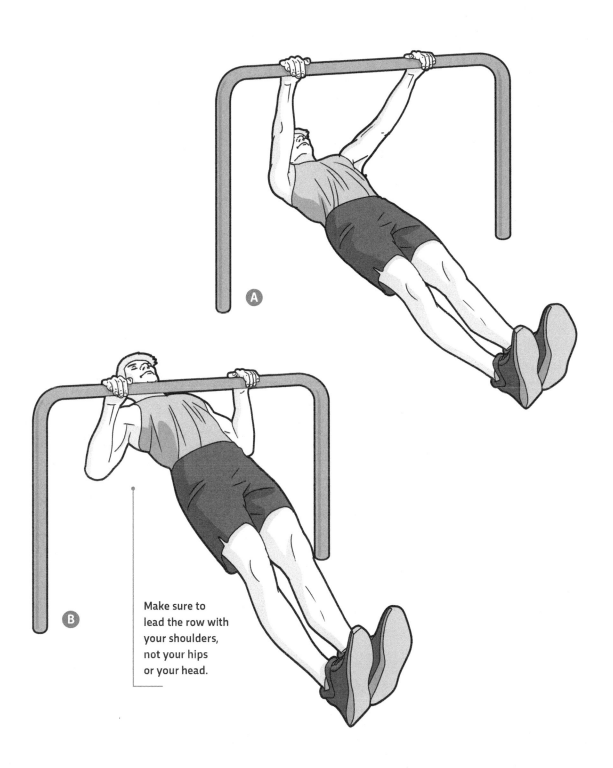

A

B

Make sure to lead the row with your shoulders, not your hips or your head.

66 / ONE ARM OPEN GRIP ROW

This variation gets difficult quickly, challenging single arm strength as well as hip and shoulder stability. Ideally, you should do this row from a higher bar so that it's not too difficult, but you can also regress it by bending your knees if your choice of bars is limited. For an extra challenge, you can add a rotation at the bottom of the row, introducing some chest and abdominals to a movement that normally focuses on your shoulders, back, and arms.

GOAL: 10 repetitions on each side

1 Grip your chosen bar with your palms facing away from you, and hang back into straight arms. Straighten your legs, dig your heels into the ground, and flex your feet so that your toes point up toward your face.

2 Make sure your left hand is lined up with your shoulder, and let go of the bar with your right hand. **A**

3 Engage your trapezius muscles by pulling your shoulders down toward your hips, retracting your shoulder blades to find stability in your shoulders. Pull your chest toward the bar by bending your left arm and pulling back your shoulder blade, being careful not to elevate your shoulder. Keeping your free right arm straight, pass it over the top of the bar. **B**

4 Once the bar touches your lower chest, slowly lower your body back to the shoulder-packed position, being careful not to extend the shoulders too far. See tip for additional rotation. **C**

5 Do the desired number of reps on the left side before switching to the right.

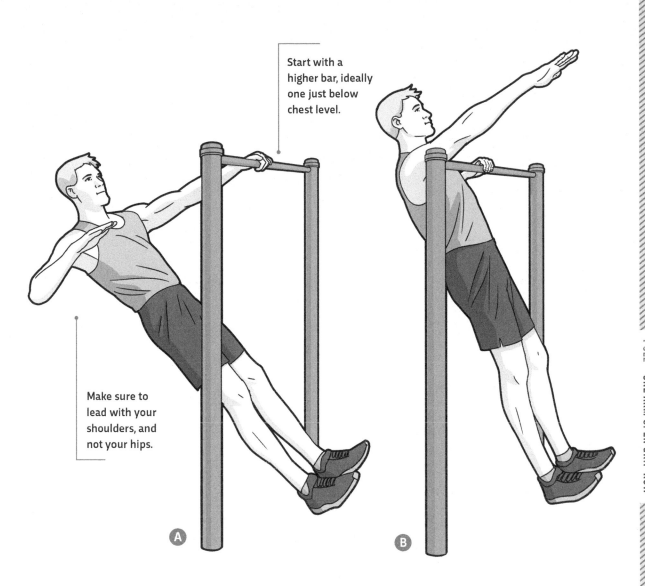

Start with a higher bar, ideally one just below chest level.

Make sure to lead with your shoulders, and not your hips.

A

B

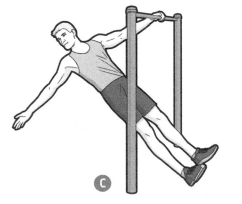

Add a rotation after step 5 by turning slowly, reaching for the ground with your free hand.

C

CLOSED GRIP PULL-UP

Primary muscle groups: Biceps, Lats
Secondary muscle group: Trapezius

67
BASE

**FLEXED
ARM HANG**

68
INTERMEDIATE

CHIN-UP

69
ADVANCED

**CHIN-UP
WITH PIKE**

Chin-ups are a type of pull-up that are executed with a closed grip, and thus the official name for them is closed grip pull-up. They typically feel a little easier than the classic pull-up because with your palms facing upward, your biceps have a more direct line of pull and can pitch in more. Rather than using a negative chin-up as a regression for this exercise, you'll start with a flexed arm hang, which is a great exercise for building shoulder stability. The second variation is the classic chin-up, and the last is a chin-up with the legs straight out in a pike position.

67 / FLEXED ARM HANG

This variation helps you develop the shoulder stability you need for proper chin-ups and pull-ups. It's a great option for building the strength necessary for a chin-up—but still a great challenge if you already have that strength. You can do it from a lower bar or from a high bar with a step under it—anything that lets you comfortably get yourself into the fully flexed position with your feet in the air. This exercise doesn't involve repetitions, so you'll aim to hold it for a certain length of time instead of counting reps.

GOAL: Your first goal should be to hold the position for intervals totaling 30 seconds. As you get stronger, progress to intervals totaling 60 seconds.

1 Using a low bar or a step beneath a high bar, position your body at the top range of a chin-up. Your elbows should be bent, and the bar should be even with or just below your chin. **A**

2 Hold the position for at least 10 seconds, making sure your shoulders stay down.

3 To release, lower yourself smoothly back to the ground or the step.

4 Jump back up or use the step to return to the starting position, and repeat.

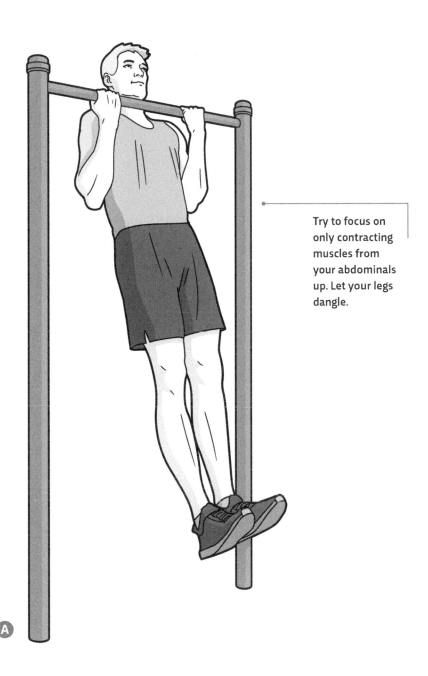

Try to focus on
only contracting
muscles from
your abdominals
up. Let your legs
dangle.

A

68 / CHIN-UP

The chin-up is a version of a pull-up that uses a closed or supinated grip (palms up) instead of a pronated one (palms down). It typically feels easier than the classic pull-up because the position of your hands allows your biceps to be more involved. Try to keep your body stable and avoid swaying back and forth as you perform the pull. This helps train your lats to fully extend without pulling your back into extension and throwing your body into a swing.

GOAL: Build up to 20 repetitions.

1 Start by hanging from a bar with your palms facing toward you. Engage your abdominals to prevent excessive extension in your lower back.

2 Keeping your shoulders depressed, pull yourself up **A** until your chin is at the same level as the bar. **B** Slowly lower yourself back into your starting position.

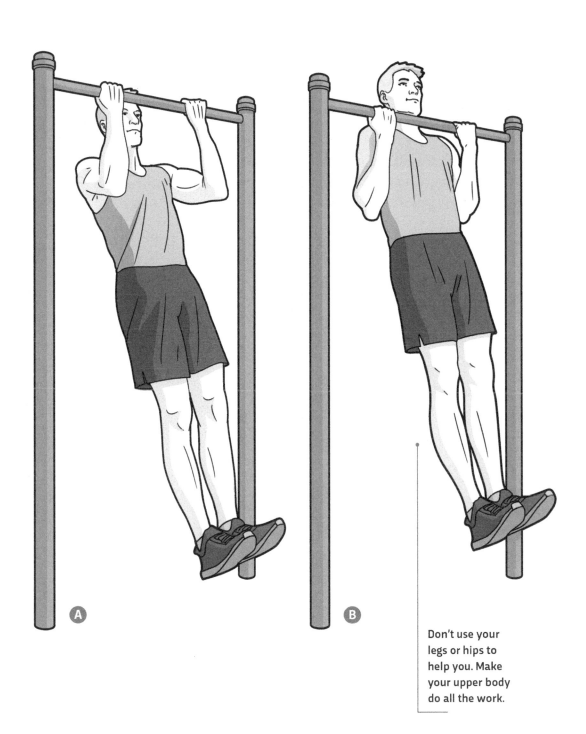

A

B

Don't use your legs or hips to help you. Make your upper body do all the work.

69 / CHIN-UP WITH PIKE

This variation of the chin-up forces your abdominals to maintain a straight-leg position through the entire motion, which prevents your lower spine from extending as a result of weak core stabilizers. It also forces your lats to fully extend at the bottom so they can't try to cheat and stay short, pulling your lower back into extension.

GOAL: 20 repetitions

1 Start by hanging from a bar with your palms facing toward you.

----

2 Engage your abdominals, and lift your legs straight out in front of you in a pike position. **A**

----

3 Keeping your shoulders depressed, pull yourself up until your chin is at bar level. **B** Slowly lower yourself back into your starting position. **A**

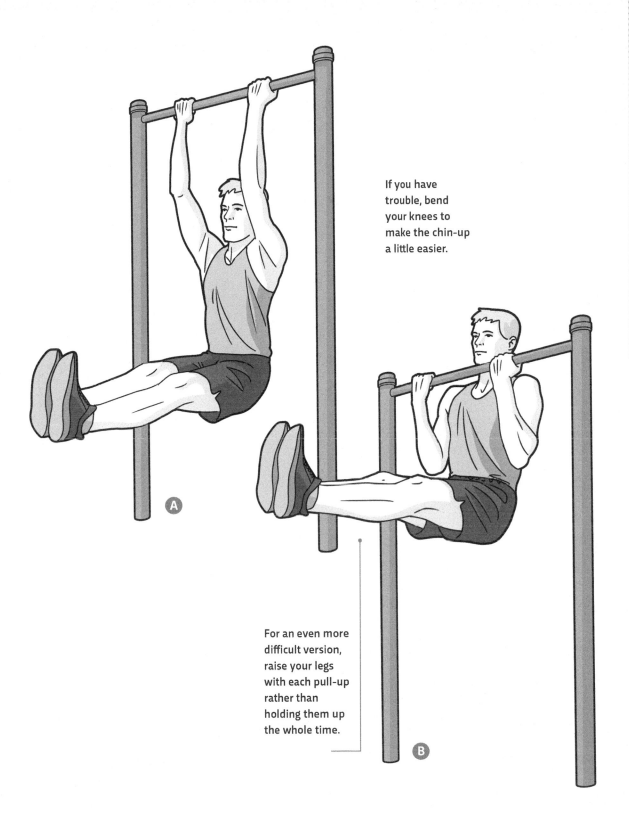

If you have trouble, bend your knees to make the chin-up a little easier.

For an even more difficult version, raise your legs with each pull-up rather than holding them up the whole time.

A

B

OPEN GRIP PULL-UP

Primary muscle groups: Biceps, Lats
Secondary muscle group: Trapezius

70
BASE

**NEGATIVE
PULL-UP**

71
INTERMEDIATE

**OPEN GRIP
PULL-UP**

72
ADVANCED

**ROCK CLIMBER
PULL-UP**

Pull-ups may just be the most difficult bodyweight exercise—but they're also the best display of total bodyweight strength. Because we rarely do this motion in our daily lives, these muscles can begin to lose strength and connection with the brain. That's why it's so important to keep your body moving through all the different ranges of motion on a regular basis. If you don't, the strength you need for rarer motions starts to disappear. The first variation of this exercise will be to lower yourself in what's called an eccentric, or negative, pull-up. The next level is a true pull-up, and the last has a horizontal shift challenge.

70 / NEGATIVE PULL-UP

For the negative pull-up, you'll want either a lower bar (head- to chest-level) or a step underneath a normal pull-up bar. You need to be able to comfortably get your body into the finishing position of a pull-up—the part where you're holding your weight up and the bar is below your chin—and then slowly lower yourself in a controlled manner until your arms are fully extended. It's like a reverse or "negative" version of a regular pull-up, where you focus on carefully lowering your body instead of lifting it. Make sure you keep your shoulders pulled down toward your hips, and don't let them ride up around your ears throughout the whole lowering motion. This will help train your lower-trapezius muscles to activate and support your shoulder blades.

GOAL: Once you can do 20 repetitions, you're ready to tackle the classic Open Grip Pull-Up (71).

1 Using a low bar or a step underneath a high bar, position your body at the top range of a pull-up. A Your elbows should be bent, and the bar should be below your chin.

2 Keeping your lower-trapezius muscles engaged by pulling your shoulders down toward your hips, slowly extend your arms, lowering your body B until your elbows are straight. C

3 Jump back up or use the step to return to the starting position, A and repeat.

230   THE ESQUIRE GUIDE TO BODYWEIGHT TRAINING

For an extra challenge, try shifting back and forth at the top of the pull-up.

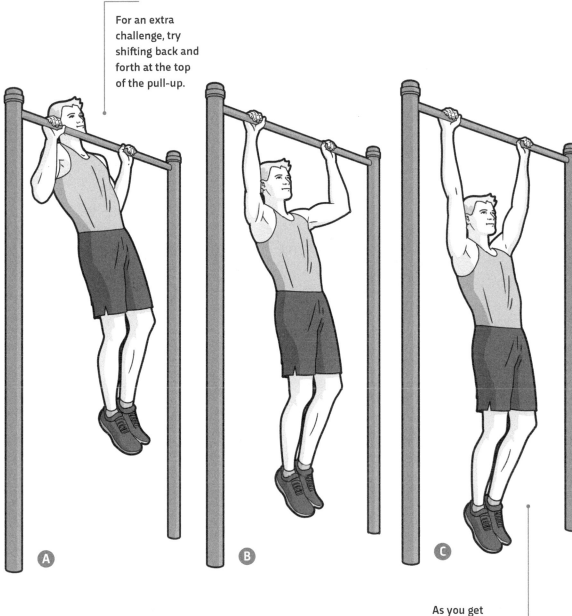

A

B

C

As you get stronger, start your set with as many pull-ups as you can do and finish the set with negatives.

71 / OPEN GRIP PULL-UP

Here it is: the true test of bodyweight strength. In this variation, you'll start from a fully extended arm position, hanging from a bar. In a good pull-up, your chin breaks the plane of the bar (without tilting your head back to get another inch or two of chin height). You don't need to go to a full dead hang between repetitions unless you want the extra challenge, but your elbows should come within just a few degrees of being straight. Make sure to keep your lower-trapezius muscles and abs firing through all phases of this exercise.

GOAL: Build up to 20 repetitions.

1 Start by hanging from a bar with your palms facing away from you. **A**

2 Engage your abdominals to prevent excessive extension in your lower back.

3 Keeping your shoulders depressed, pull yourself up **B** until your chin is at the bar's level. **C** Slowly lower yourself back into your starting position. **A**

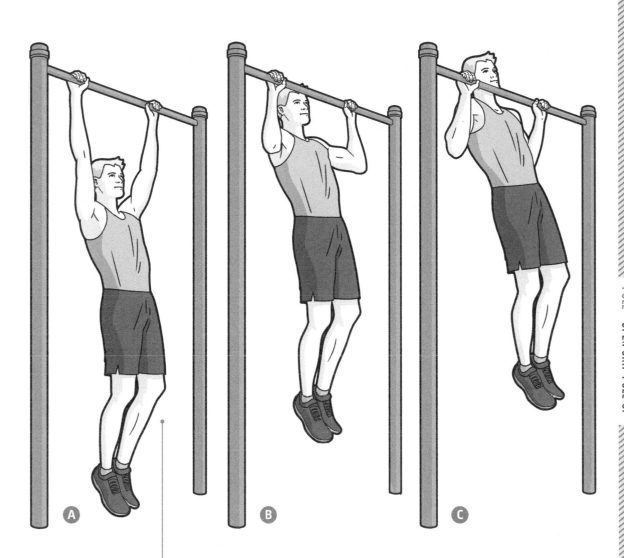

You can bend your knees to lighten the load on your abdominals, but don't let your lower back go into hyperextension.

72 / ROCK CLIMBER PULL-UP

These pull-ups take your body from one side to another, alternately challenging each side to do more of the pulling. Your goal is to get your right shoulder to tap your right hand as you pull up to your right side, and then do the same on the left. As you go up and down, try to keep your lateral translation smooth, and match it with your vertical motion. The wider your hand grip, the harder this variation will be.

GOAL: 10 repetitions on each side

1 Start by hanging from a bar with your palms facing away from you.

----

2 Engage your abdominals to prevent excessive extension in your lower back.

----

3 Keeping your shoulders depressed, pull your right shoulder up to your right hand. **A**

----

4 Lower yourself smoothly back into your starting position. Repeat on the left side. **B**

To make the move a little easier, you can bring your hands closer together to lessen your lateral shift.

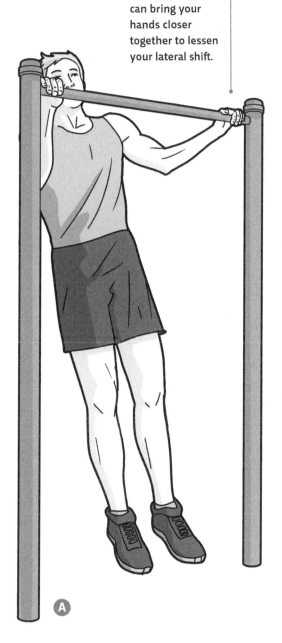

A

For an extra challenge, try shifting back and forth at the top of the pull-up.

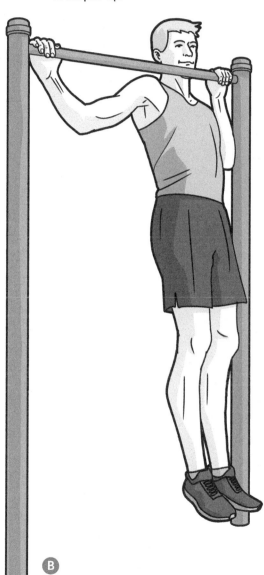

B

235

SPINAL EXTENSION

Primary muscle groups: Spinal erectors, Trapezius
Secondary muscle group: Deltoids

73
BASE

PRONE
SPINAL
EXTENSION

74
INTERMEDIATE

PRONE
SWIMMER

75
ADVANCED

PRONE
SHOULDER
PRESS

Spinal extensions are great for strengthening your mid-spine extensors and activating your mid and lower-trapezius muscles, which control your shoulder blades. Building good rhythm between your shoulder blades and your arms is essential for healthy arm and shoulder movement. It's important to practice correct depression and retraction of your shoulder blades so that your upper trapezius muscles don't become overactive when your arms are overhead. These exercises are a great way to build that control. Begin each exercise lying face down, which is known as the prone position.

73 / PRONE SPINAL EXTENSION

The most basic of the spinal extensions, this exercise involves lifting your head, shoulders, and chest off the ground while leaving your legs and hips neutral and in contact with the ground. It doesn't use repetitions, so, like you did with the flexed arm hang (67), you'll aim to hold it for a certain length of time. Try to keep your shoulders rolled open into outward rotation and your elbows lower than your wrists.

GOAL: **Start by holding the position for intervals totaling 30 seconds. Progress to intervals totaling 60 and then 90 seconds.**

1 Lie face down. Your hands should be palms down, placed even with, and just wider than, your shoulders.

---

2 Make sure your shoulder blades are pressed down toward your hips and slightly retracted.

---

3 Gently lift your head, shoulders, and arms a few inches off the ground as one unit. **Ⓐ** The movement should come from the middle of your spine with the lower spine staying relatively relaxed.

---

4 Hold this position for 30 seconds, breathing deeply and trying to get your chest taller and the back of your neck longer with each exhalation.

If you have difficulty, stretch out your pectoral muscles and middle spine first with the supine pec stretch (page 259).

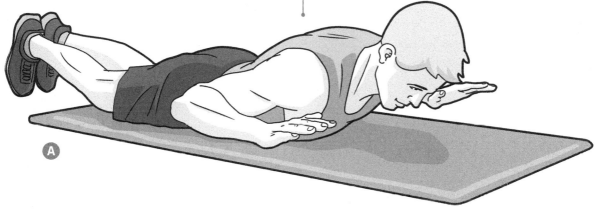

A

74 / PRONE SWIMMER

This variation begins to challenge the upward and downward rotation of your shoulder blades (scapulae) as you reach your arms overhead. The point of this exercise is to work your shoulders' outward rotators and to practice moving your arms overhead without allowing the upper traps to become overactive. Your shoulders should not creep up around your ears. If you can't get your arms all the way up over your head without using your upper-trapezius muscles, only go as high as you can. Move your arms in an alternating pattern, and focus on returning them to a low position that lets your upper-trapezius muscles completely turn off between each rep.

GOAL: 20 repetitions

1 Lie face down. Your hands should be palms down, placed even with, and just wider than, your shoulders.

----

2 Make sure your shoulder blades are pressed down toward your hips and slightly retracted.

----

3 Gently lift your head, shoulders, and arms a few inches off the ground as one unit. **A** The movement should come from your middle spine, while your lower spine stays relaxed.

----

4 Keeping your arms and hands just an inch from the ground, slowly reach one arm overhead, **A** trying to straighten your elbow while preventing overactivity of your upper trapezius muscles.

----

5 As you return that arm to the starting position, extend the other in a reciprocating motion. **B**

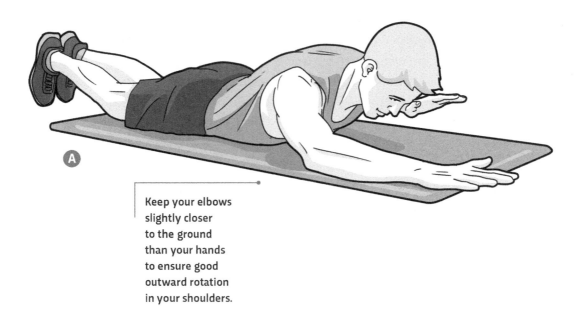

Keep your elbows slightly closer to the ground than your hands to ensure good outward rotation in your shoulders.

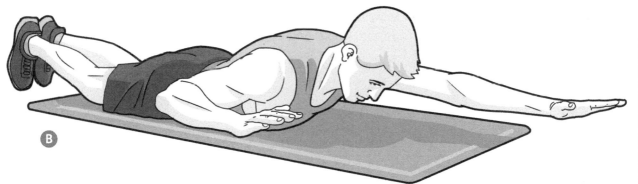

75 / PRONE SHOULDER PRESS

The prone shoulder press is similar to the prone swimmer (74), but this one challenges motion in both shoulder blades at the same time. Moving one side of your body at a time involves different mechanics than moving both sides together, and you may find this variation more difficult. Remember, only bring your arms as high overhead as you can before your upper-trapezius muscles kick in. You want to keep your lower- and mid-trapezius muscles engaged and keep your upper-trapezius muscles from becoming overactive. You should not feel stress in your neck while doing this exercise. If you do, you need to strive for more lower-trapezius engagement and more outward rotation of your shoulders and arms. Also check to make sure you're not craning your neck and trying to look out in front of you.

GOAL: 20 repetitions

1 Lie face down. Your hands should be palms down, placed even with, and just wider than, your shoulders. Make sure your shoulder blades are pressed down toward your hips and slightly retracted.

------

2 Gently lift your head, shoulders, and arms a few inches off the ground as one unit. Ⓐ The movement should come from your middle spine, while your lower spine stays relaxed.

------

3 Keeping your arms and hands just an inch from the ground, slowly reach up overhead with both hands, straightening your elbows as best you can. Ⓑ

------

4 Return to the starting position as soon as you feel your upper trapezius muscles starting to pull your shoulders up toward your ears or your elbows lifting up.

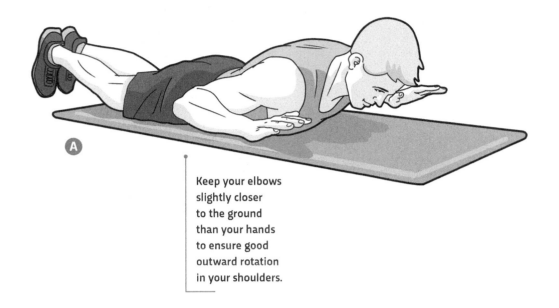

A

Keep your elbows
slightly closer
to the ground
than your hands
to ensure good
outward rotation
in your shoulders.

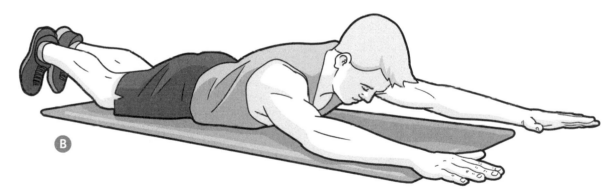

B

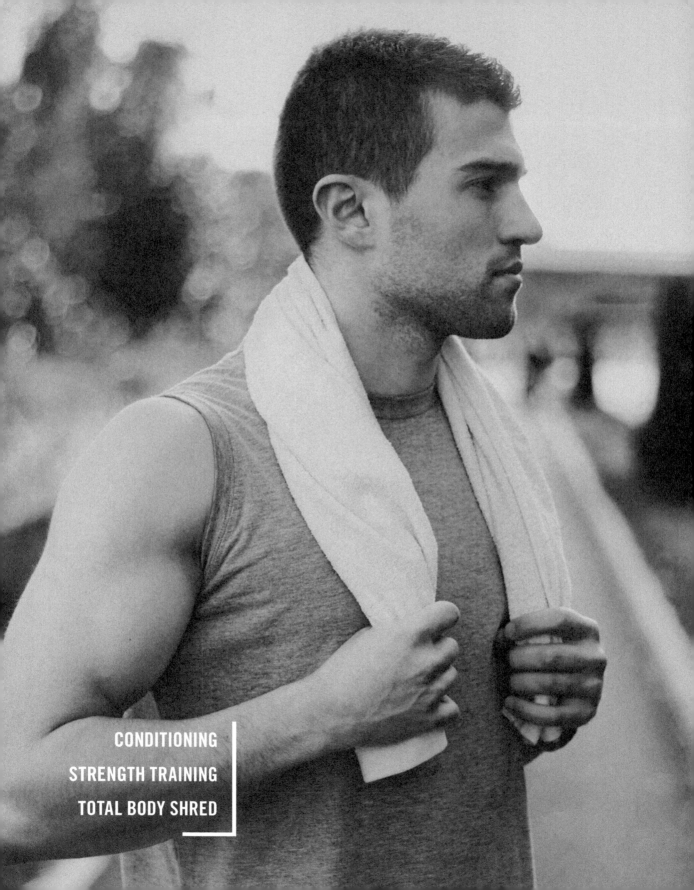

CONDITIONING

STRENGTH TRAINING

TOTAL BODY SHRED

EIGHT

THE WORKOUT PROGRAMS

Push-ups, pull-ups, lunges, squats. These exercises aren't exactly surprising or new to you. What makes them so powerful is that, when combined into a single workout, they offer an efficient and intense full-body session unlike anything else. And that starts here.

This section of the book offers three different programs: Conditioning (4 weeks), Strength Training (8 weeks), and Total Body Shred (12 weeks).

The programs consist of several types of workout structures. Some are full body and work every movement category, while others are like a yin and yang to each other, balancing pushes with pulls, horizontal movements with vertical ones, and hip-driven movements with ankle-driven ones. These workouts have been designed and ordered to make sure your workouts are balanced over the course of the program and to help you achieve well-proportioned results.

Here's what you'll see in each workout:

COLOR: Each workout is identified by a different color (purple, blue, or green) for easy reference in the programming.

TEMPO: The speed at which you perform a rep. Tempo is written in terms of seconds up or down. In the context of a squat, for example, *1 second up* means taking 1 second to come up from a squat and *1 second down* means taking 1 second to drop down to the bottom of a squat.

REPS: The number of times to repeat an exercise before starting a rest interval.

All repetition schemes in these workouts are broken up into 10, 15, and 20 reps for you to choose from, depending on your ability. This is a simple variable you can use as a progression and/or a way to track change in your performance. Some of these exercises will be really difficult to get through with 20 repetitions, so start with

10 or 15 and work your way up. Keep in mind that you don't have to stay consistent on repetitions through a whole circuit. If one exercise is limiting you to 10 repetitions, you can still go for 15 or 20 with all the others.

REST INTERVAL: The amount of time you can take between exercises for recovery.

WORK:REST: A ratio between performing an exercise and recovery. Written in seconds, this will look something like 30:45, meaning for every active 30 seconds, rest for 45 seconds. This appears in the workouts in Program Three only.

CIRCUIT: A group of exercises that should be done in order and succession before returning to the first exercise. Some workouts have one long circuit while others have two shorter ones. The number that appears, followed by an X, indicates the number of times to go through each circuit.

EXERCISE NAME: The exercise name is immediately followed by the the exercise's number in the book (1–75). This is *not* the page number on which you'll find the exercise.

Injuries and imbalances in the body can make getting results from a fitness program difficult to impossible. Mobility exercises should be an integral part of any well-planned workout regimen and are essential to reaching your potential. Turn to page 257 to find six mobility cooldown poses. At the end of each workout, choose at least three from the list, if not more, and relax, allowing your muscles to stretch out.

PROGRAM ONE
CONDITIONING

---

4 WEEKS

This program is meant to introduce bodyweight training movements and is perfect for beginners. Each day is a fully balanced workout, so you don't need to worry about balancing one type of workout with another type later in the week. It initially focuses on the base level of each exercise but progresses to the more advanced versions later in the program.

WORKOUT WEEK		MONDAY	TUESDAY	WEDNESDAY	THURSDAY	FRIDAY	SATURDAY	SUNDAY
	1	A	Rest	B	Rest	A	Rest	B
	2	Rest	C	D	Rest	C	D	Rest
	3	A	D	Rest	B	C	Rest	D
	4	C	B	Rest	D	A	B	Rest

A

Tempo
1 sec ↑ and ↓

Reps
10/15/20

Rest Interval
30 seconds

Circuit
3X

Squat (19)

Elevated push-up (46)

Negative pull-up (70)

Two leg hip hinge (43)

Bent knee
bench dip (58)

Bent knee closed
grip row (61)

Forward bear
crawl (04)

B

Tempo
1 sec ↑ and ↓

Reps
10/15/20

Rest Interval
30 seconds

Circuit
3X

Reverse lunge (22)

Horizontal sliding
push-up from
knees (49)

Flexed arm hang (67)
hold for 30/60 sec

Floor bridge (34)

Bent knee pike
push-up (52)

Bent knee open
grip row (64)

Classic plank (01)
hold for 30/60 sec

C

Tempo
1 sec ↑ and ↓

Reps
10/15/20

Rest Interval
30 seconds

Circuit
3X

Forward step-up (25)

Elevated push-up (46)

Negative pull-up (70)

Quadruped
straight tap (41)

Bent knee
bench dip (58)

Bent knee closed
grip row (61)

Supine leg raise (13)

D

Tempo
1 sec ↑ and ↓

Reps
10/15/20

Rest Interval
30 seconds

Circuit
3X

Walking lunge (23)

Elevated push-up (46)

Flexed arm hang (67)
hold for 30/60 sec

Staggered
hip hinge (44)

Bent knee pike
push-up (52)

Bent knee open
grip row (64)

Side plank (02)
hold for 30/60 sec

PROGRAM TWO
STRENGTH TRAINING

8 WEEKS

This program focuses on building strength. If you're a beginner, start it after completing Program One. If you're more physically active, you can try it out right away. It has fewer rest days and a slower repetition tempo. Note that each workout in this program consists of two different circuits, both focusing on similar exercise categories. Circuit One should be completed four times before moving to Circuit Two.

	MONDAY	TUESDAY	WEDNESDAY	THURSDAY	FRIDAY	SATURDAY	SUNDAY
1	A	B	*Rest*	A	B	*Rest*	C
2	D	*Rest*	C	D	*Rest*	A	B
3	C	*Rest*	D	A	D	*Rest*	C
4	D	C	*Rest*	B	C	D	*Rest*
5	E	F	G	G	*Rest*	E	F
6	G	H	*Rest*	C	E	H	*Rest*
7	B	C	G	F	*Rest*	E	L
8	A	*Rest*	G	F	L	E	*Rest*

(WORKOUT WEEK)

A

Tempo
2 sec ↓ and 1 sec ↑

Repetitions
10/15/20

Rest Interval
30 seconds

Circuit
4X through each

CIRCUIT ONE

Squat (19)

Classic push-up (47)

Negative pull-up (70)

Forward bear
crawl (04)

CIRCUIT TWO

Reverse lunge (22)

T push-up (55)

Flexed arm hang (67)
hold for 30/60 sec

Side plank (02)
hold for 30/60 sec

B

Tempo
2 sec ↓ and 1 sec ↑

Repetitions
10/15/20

Rest Interval
30 seconds

Circuit
4X through each

CIRCUIT ONE

Two leg hip hinge (43)

Bent knee pike
push-up (52)

Bent knee open
grip row (64)

Classic plank (01)
hold for 30/60 sec

CIRCUIT TWO

One leg floor
bridge (35)

Bent knee
bench dip (58)

Bent knee closed
grip row (61)

Supine leg raise (13)

C

Tempo
2 sec ↓ and 1 sec ↑

Repetitions
10/15/20

Rest Interval
30 seconds

Circuit
4X through each

CIRCUIT ONE

Walking lunge (23)

Push-up with
shoulder tap (48)

Chin-up (68)

Bicycle (10)

CIRCUIT TWO

Side lunge (24)

Horizontal sliding
push-up from
knees (49)

Negative pull-up (70)

Lateral crab walk (05)

D

Tempo
2 sec ↓ and 1 sec ↑

Repetitions
10/15/20

Rest Interval
30 seconds

Circuit
4X through each

CIRCUIT ONE

Shoulder-elevated
bridge (37)

Straight leg
bench dip (59)

Straight leg closed
grip row (62)

Plank walk-up (03)

CIRCUIT TWO

Staggered hip
hinge (44)

Bent knee pike
push-up (52)

Straight leg open
grip row (64)

Plank with rotational
knee tuck (15)

E

Tempo
2 sec ↓ and 1 sec ↑

Repetitions
10/15/20

Rest Interval
30 seconds

Circuit
4X through each

CIRCUIT ONE

Forward step-up (25)

Straight-leg
bench dip (59)

Chin-up (68)

Windshield wiper (11)
(with bent knees)

CIRCUIT TWO

Squat (19)

Bent knee pike
push-up (52)

Prone swimmer (74)

Hanging leg raise (14)

F

Tempo
2 sec ↓ and 1 sec ↑

Repetitions
10/15/20

Rest Interval
30 seconds

Circuit
4X through each

CIRCUIT ONE

One leg hip hinge (45)

Vertical sliding
push-up (51)

Bent knee closed
grip row (61)

Side plank (02)
hold for 30/60 sec

CIRCUIT TWO

Quadruped
straight tap (41)

Side-to-side
push-up (56)

One arm open
grip row (66)

Glanimal crawl (06)

G

Tempo
2 sec ↓ and 1 sec ↑

Repetitions
10/15/20

Rest Interval
30 seconds

Circuit
4X through each

CIRCUIT ONE

Reverse lunge (22)

Dip (59–60) parallel
bar or straight leg
bench

Rock climber
pull-up (72)

Plank walk-up (03)

CIRCUIT TWO

Side lunge (24)

Bent knee pike
push-up (52)

Prone swimmer (74)

Windshield wiper (11)

H

Tempo
2 sec ↓ and 1 sec ↑

Repetitions
10/15/20

Rest Interval
30 seconds

Circuit
4X through each

CIRCUIT ONE

One arm shoulder-
elevated bridge (39)

Scooping push-up (57)

Switch grip row (63)

Plank with rotational
kick-through (12)

CIRCUIT TWO

One leg hip hinge (45)

Push-up with
shoulder tap (48)

One arm open
grip row (66)

Forward bear
crawl (04)

PROGRAM THREE
TOTAL BODY SHRED

12 WEEKS

This plan is for people who've tried the conditioning and strength programs and are ready for something more. It circulates between conditioning workouts that focus on time rather than repetition and strength workouts with high intensity intervals built in. When you see a work-to-rest ratio listed instead of repetitions, it means you should do as many reps as you can during the work period and recover during the rest period. So if you were doing squats and your work-to-rest ratio was 15:30, you'd do as many squats as possible for 15 seconds, and then rest for 30 seconds before moving on to the next exercise.

WORKOUT WEEK	MONDAY	TUESDAY	WEDNESDAY	THURSDAY	FRIDAY	SATURDAY	SUNDAY
1	A	B	C	*Rest*	D	E	F
2	*Rest*	I	J	*Rest*	K	L	*Rest*
3	I	A	L	*Rest*	J	B	K
4	*Rest*	G	L	K	H	*Rest*	C
5	J	I	D	*Rest*	M	N	O
6	P	*Rest*	A	B	E	F	*Rest*
7	C	D	G	H	*Rest*	M	B
8	F	N	*Rest*	O	E	A	P
9	*Rest*	I	J	K	L	*Rest*	P
10	O	N	M	*Rest*	G	P	H
11	M	C	*Rest*	D	N	E	O
12	F	*Rest*	G	A	H	B	*Rest*

A	B	C	D
Tempo 1 sec ↑ and ↓	**Tempo** 1 sec ↑ and ↓	**Tempo** 1 sec ↑ and ↓	**Tempo** 1 sec ↑ and ↓
Work:Rest 15:30, 30:45, or 30:30	**Work:Rest** 15:30, 30:45, or 30:30	**Work:Rest** 15:30, 30:45, or 30:30	**Work:Rest** 15:30, 30:45, or 30:30
Circuit 4X	**Circuit** 4X	**Circuit** 4X	**Circuit** 4X
Squat (19)	Two leg hip hinge (43)	Walking lunge (23)	Shoulder-elevated bridge (37)
Classic push-up (47)	Bent knee pike push-up (52)	Push-up with shoulder tap (48)	Straight leg bench dip (59)
Negative pull-up (70)	Bent knee open grip row (64)	Chin-up (68)	Straight leg closed grip row (62)
Forward bear crawl (04)	Power bound (33)	Classic burpee (17)	One leg power jump (30)
Broad jump (32)	Reverse lunge (22)	Staggered hip hinge (44)	Side lunge (24)
Bent knee bench dip (58)	T push-up (55)	Bent knee pike push-up (52)	Horizontal sliding push-up from feet (50)
Bent knee closed grip row (61)	Flexed arm hang (67)	Straight leg open grip row (65)	Negative pull-up (70)
Supine leg raise (13)	Side plank (02)	Plank with rotational knee tuck (15)	Lateral crab walk (05)

E

Tempo
1 sec ↑ and ↓

Work:Rest
15:30, 30:45, or 30:30

Circuit
4X

Rear elevated split squat (21)

Bent knee pike push-up (52)

Prone swimmer (74)

Elevated burpee (16)

One leg hip hinge (45)

Classic push-up (47)

Straight leg closed grip row (62)

Plank walk-up (03)

F

Tempo
1 sec ↑ and ↓

Work:Rest
15:30, 30:45, or 30:30

Circuit
4X

Forward step-up (25)

Straight leg bench dip (59)

Chin-up (68)

Box jump (29)

Quadruped oblique tap (42)

Side to side push-up (56)

One arm open grip row (66)

Glanimal crawl (06)

G

Tempo
1 sec ↑ and ↓

Work:Rest
15:30, 30:45, or 30:30

Circuit
4X

Reverse lunge (22)

Dip (59–60)
parallel bar or straight leg bench

Rock climber pull-up (72)

Power bound (33)

One leg hip hinge (45)

Push-up with shoulder tap (48)

One arm open grip row (66)

Windshield wiper (11)

H

Tempo
1 sec ↑ and ↓

Work:Rest
15:30, 30:45, or 30:30

Circuit
4X

Side lunge (24)

Bent knee pike push-up (52)

Prone swimmer (74)

Broad jump (32)

One arm shoulder-elevated bridge (39)

Scooping push-up (57)

Switch grip row (63)

Plank with rotational kick-through (12)

I

Tempo
1 sec ↑ and ↓

Work:Rest
15:30, 30:45, or 30:30

Circuit
3X

Split squat (20)

T push-up (55)

Open grip pull-up (71)

Ice skater (31)

Reverse lunge (22)

Vertical sliding
push-up (51)

Flexed arm hang (67)
hold for 30/60 sec

Lateral crab walk (05)

J

Tempo
1 sec ↑ and ↓

Repetitions
10/15/20

Rest Interval
30 seconds

Circuit
3X through each

CIRCUIT ONE

One leg hip hinge (45)

Straight leg bench
dip (59) feet-elevated

Straight leg closed
grip row (62)

Forward bear
crawl (04)

CIRCUIT TWO

Floor bridge (34)

Straight leg pike
push-up (53)

Straight leg open
grip row (65)

Floor jump (28)

K

Tempo
1 sec ↑ and ↓

Repetitions
10/15/20

Rest Interval
30 seconds

Circuit
3X through each

CIRCUIT ONE

Transverse
step-up (26)

Side to side
push-up (56)

Negative pull-up (70)

Classic burpee (17)

CIRCUIT TWO

Walking lunge (23)

Elevated push-up (46)

Flexed arm hang (67)
hold for 30/60 sec

Plank with rotational
kick-through (12)

L

Tempo
1 sec ↑ and ↓

Repetitions
10/15/20

Rest Interval
30 seconds

Circuit
3X through each

CIRCUIT ONE

Staggered hip
hinge (44)

Bent-knee pike
push-up (52)

Straight leg
open-grip row (65)

Side plank (02)
hold for 30/60 sec

CIRCUIT TWO

Quadruped
oblique tap (42)

Straight leg
bench dip (59)

Bent knee closed
grip row (61)

Broad jump (32)

M

Tempo
1 sec ↑ and ↓

Repetitions
10/15/20

Rest Interval
30 seconds

Circuit
3X through each

CIRCUIT ONE

Transverse
step-up (26)

Straight leg pike
push-up (53)

Prone swimmer (74)

Plank walk-up (03)

CIRCUIT TWO

Reverse lunge (22)

Straight leg
bench dip (59)

Chin-up (68)

Power bound (33)

N

Tempo
1 sec ↑ and ↓

Repetitions
10/15/20

Rest Interval
30 seconds

Circuit
3X through each

CIRCUIT ONE

One leg hip hinge (45)

Push-up with
shoulder tap (48)

Bent knee closed
grip row (61)

Forward bear
crawl (04)

CIRCUIT TWO

Floor bridge (34)

T push-up (55)

One-arm open grip
row (66)

Ice skater (31)

O

Tempo
1 sec ↑ and ↓

Repetitions
10/15/20

Rest Interval
30 seconds

Circuit
3X through each

CIRCUIT ONE

Transverse
step-up (26)

Handstand
push-up (54)

Flexed arm hang (67)
hold for 30/60 sec

Elevated burpee (16)

CIRCUIT TWO

Walking lunge (23)

Prone shoulder
press (75)

Negative pull-up (70)

One leg power
jump (30)

P

Tempo
1 sec ↑ and ↓

Repetitions
10/15/20

Rest Interval
30 seconds

Circuit
3X through each

CIRCUIT ONE

Staggered hip
hinge (44)

Scooping push-up (57)

Straight leg open
grip row (65)

Side plank (02)
hold for 30/60 sec

CIRCUIT TWO

Quadruped
oblique tap (42)

Elevated push-up (46)

Bent knee closed
grip row (61)

One arm burpee (18)

MOBILITY COOLDOWN

6 POSTWORKOUT POSES

Use these mobility exercises as a cooldown. The goal is to achieve relaxation, rather than put extreme tension on a muscle and try to hold it for as long as you can. When your muscles are warm, they are more flexible. After a workout, it's as if your muscles are like molten rock. The idea is to allow them to cool down in the following poses, which encourages them to "harden" with more length in their resting state. ■ Pick two or three of these poses for your cooldown, and try to hold each for two to three minutes, coming in and out of them as needed. Do not overdo these if you have difficulty. Ease in and practice them gently. Listen to your body, and remember that relaxation is the goal, not enduring discomfort for as long as possible.

KNEELING WITH FEET FLAT OUT

Helps to regain and maintain functional mobility in the ankles. ■ Allows the low back and pelvis to relax in a neutral position.

Let your heels fall out and help train the ankle to allow external rotation of the shin bone.

If you are uncomfortable putting your full weight on your ankles, you can lean forward to distribute some weight into your hands.

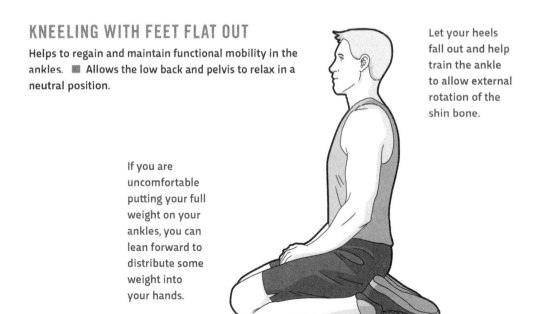

KNEELING WITH TOES TUCKED UNDER

Helps stretch the plantar fascia on the bottom of the foot, promoting malleability, as well as foot and arch functionality.

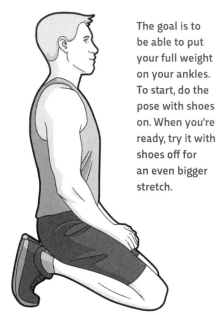

The goal is to be able to put your full weight on your ankles. To start, do the pose with shoes on. When you're ready, try it with shoes off for an even bigger stretch.

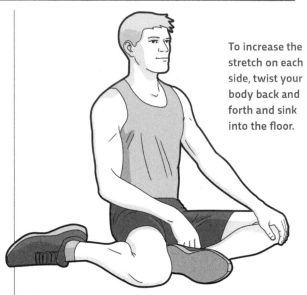

To increase the stretch on each side, twist your body back and forth and sink into the floor.

SIDESADDLE

Works to rotate the hips internally and externally for healthier movement patterns. Proper internal and external rotation of the hip has the potential to greatly reduce lower back pain. If you can't sit comfortably, feel free to put some weight into one of your hands.

HALF KNEELING

Allows the hip to rest in a neutral or slightly extended position by tilting the top of the pelvis backward, which elongates the hip flexor and builds pelvic tilt control. ■ Allow the down leg heel to fall out, which encourages external rotation of the shin bone, promoting healthy forward movement of the shin over the foot in ankle-driven exercises.

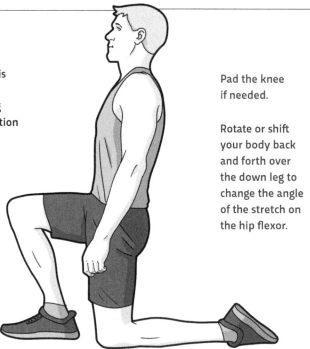

Pad the knee if needed.

Rotate or shift your body back and forth over the down leg to change the angle of the stretch on the hip flexor.

FULL SQUAT

Trains maximum flexion of the hips and promotes healthy forward movement of the shin over the foot. The goal is feet parallel but, if that's too challenging, start by turning them out to widen your foot base. Make sure arches do not collapse.

■ As you get better, practice lifting your chest taller. When you're ready, challenge the extension of your midback by trying to put your hands behind your head.

Feel free to start with an assist, like hanging onto something or putting your back against a wall.

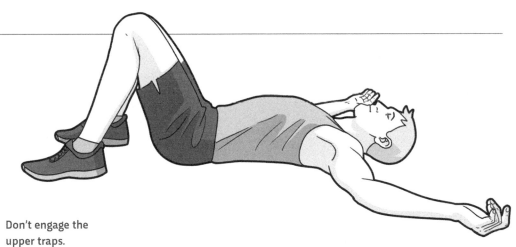

Don't engage the upper traps.

Start with the arms low and work your way up as you progress.

SUPINE PEC STRETCH

Restores a more natural midback curve and shoulder position. ■ Stretches the overtight pectorals and internal rotators of the arms and shoulders.

GLOSSARY

ABDUCTION The motion of a body part away from your body's midline.

ADDUCTION The motion of a body part toward the body's midline.

ANKLE-DRIVEN MOVEMENT Movement resulting from the dorsiflexion of the ankle, which allows the shin to move forward over the center of the foot.

ANTIROTATION Preventing rotation. Your core muscles provide antirotational stability when they keep your torso from turning.

DELTOIDS Large triangle-shaped muscles that cover the shoulder and help abduct, flex, and extend the arm.

DEPRESSION (SHOULDER MOTION) Downward movement that lowers your shoulders vertically toward your hips. Shoulder muscles depress when you do pulling exercises.

DORSIFLEXION The motion of bringing your foot up toward your shin, or, more functionally, lowering your shin toward your foot in a standing position, elongating your calf.

ELEVATION (SHOULDER MOTION) Upward movement that raises your shoulders vertically. Shrugging your shoulders is an example of elevation.

FASCIA The connective tissue that covers and binds together muscle.

FLEXIBILITY The range of motion you have in your joints in a passive state.

GLUTEAL MUSCLES A group of three muscles—gluteus maximus, gluteus medius, and gluteus minimus—that make up your buttocks. Colloquially known as "glutes," they help move and stabilize your hips.

GLYCOGEN A simple sugar, which is the stored form of carbohydrates, used for energy.

HIP-DRIVEN MOVEMENT Movement derived from the articulation of the femur (thigh bone) and pelvis.

LATISSIMUS DORSI The large muscles on either side of the midback that help you adduct your arms.

MOBILITY The range of motion you have in your joints in an active state.

PECTORALS The large muscles that cover most of your chest and help you bring your arms together.

PLANTAR FLEXION Ankle movement that flexes your foot and toes downward, shortening your calf.

PRONATE To turn the sole of your foot away from the midline of your body, or to turn your palms down toward the ground.

PROTRACTION (SHOULDER MOTION) The spreading of your shoulder blades away from each other.

RETRACTION (SHOULDER MOTION) The pulling of your shoulder blades closer together.

ROTATION Turning or rotating of your mid and upper spine. Your core muscles provide rotational motion when you turn your torso.

SUPINATE To turn the sole of your foot toward the midline of your body. To turn your palms up toward the sky.

REFERENCES

Behrens, M., A. Mau-Moeller, K. Mueller, S. Heise, M. Gube, N. Beuster, P. K. Herlyn, et al. "Plyometric Training Improves Voluntary Activation and Strength during Isometric, Concentric, and Eccentric Contractions." *Journal of Science and Medicine in Sport*. February 4, 2015. doi:10.1016/j.jsams.2015.01.011.

Breslow, Rosalind A., Chiung M. Chen, Barry I. Graubard, Tova Jacobovitz, and Ashima Kant. "Diets of Drinkers on Drinking and Nondrinking Days: NHANES 2003–2008." *American Journal of Clinical Nutrition* 97, no. 5 (May 2013): 1068–75. doi:10.3945/ajcn.112.050161.

Guinness World Records. "Most Pull-Ups in One Minute." June 15, 2015. www.guinnessworldrecords.com/world-records/most-pull-ups-in-one-minute.

Harper, Douglas. "Calisthenics." *Online Etymology Dictionary*. Accessed October 30, 2015. etymonline.com/index.php?allowed_in_frame=0&search=calisthenics&searchmode=none.

International Olympic Committee. "Factsheet: The Olympic Games of Antiquity." May 2012. www.olympic.org/documents/reference_documents_factsheets/the_olympic_games_of_the_antiquity.pdf.

Johansson, Scarlett. "The Skinny." *Huffington Post*. Last modified May 25, 2011. www.huffingtonpost.com/scarlett-johansson/the-skinny_b_186233.html.

MannyPacquiaoOfficial. "Manny Pacquiao Complete Ab Workout." YouTube. April 7, 2011. www.youtube.com/watch?v=0JN8Nque1Sc.

Melina, Remy. "Man Sets Record for Most World Records." LiveScience. May 13, 2011. www.livescience.com/14160-holder-guinness-world-records.html.

National Heart, Lung, and Blood Institute. "Larger Portion Sizes Contribute to U.S. Obesity Problem." National Institutes of Health. Last modified February 13, 2013. www.nhlbi.nih.gov/health/educational/wecan/news-events/matte1.htm.

Rodriguez-Rosell, D., F. Franco Márquez, F. Pareja-Blanco, R. Mora-Custodio, J. M. Yáñez-García, J. M. González-Suárez, and J. J. González-Badillo. "Effects of 6-Weeks Resistance Training Combined with Plyometric and Speed Exercises on Physical Performance of Pre-peak Height Velocity Soccer Players." *International Journal of Sports Physiology and Performance*. July 27, 2015. www.ncbi.nlm.nih.gov/pubmed/26218231.

Seidenberg, Casey. "Fermented Foods Bubble with Healthful Benefits." *Washington Post*. November 19, 2012. www.washingtonpost.com/blogs/on -parenting/post/fermented-foods-bubble -with-healthful-benefits/2012/11/19 /db70ea76-329b-11e2-9cfa-e41bac 906cc9_blog.html.

Smith, Dave. "13 Legit Reasons to Start Bodyweight Training Today." Greatist.com. August 12, 2015. greatist.com/fitness /start-bodyweight-training.

Thapoung, Kenny. "Cobie Smulders' 10 Smartest Quotes About Fit Living." *Women's Health*. March 26, 2014. www.womenshealthmag.com/fitness /cobie-smulders-fitness-tips.

The Tallest Man. "Angus MacAskill—7 feet 9 inches (236.2 cm)." Accessed December 8, 2015. www.thetallestman.com /angusmacaskill.htm.

Thompson, Walter R. "Worldwide Survey of Fitness Trends for 2015: What's Driving the Market." *ACSM's Health & Fitness Journal* 18, no. 6 (November/December 2014): 8–17. journals.lww.com/acsm -healthfitness/fulltext/2014/11000 /worldwide_survey_of_fitness_trends _for_2015_.5.aspx.

University of Maryland Medical Center. "Low Back Pain." Last modified January 20, 2012. umm.edu/health/medical/altmed /condition/low-back-pain.

Van Luling, Todd. "'American Ninja Warrior' Winner Challenges Show to Make Course Harder Next Time." *Huffington Post*. Last modified September 18, 2015. www.huffingtonpost.com /entry/american-ninja-warrior-winner _55fb0dd6e4b0fde8b0cd6d6c.

INDEX OF EXERCISES

INDEX

step-up
Forward Step-Up, 104–105
Transverse Step-Up, 106–107
Strength Training program,
32, 249–251
Supine Pec Stretch, 259
See also pectorals

T

tempo, 246
Total Body Shred program,
32–33, 252–256

trapezius, 19, 206–211, 214–219,
222–227, 230–235, 238–243
triceps, 19, 164–169, 172–177,
180–185, 188–193, 196–201
TRX, 18

V

vegetables, eating, 27

W

waistline, measuring, 21
water, drinking, 29

workout clothes and
accessories, 29–30
workout programs, 32–33,
245–246
Conditioning, 247–248
Strength Training, 249–251
Total Body Shred, 252–256
Work:Rest ratio, 246

ACKNOWLEDGMENTS

ABOUT THE AUTHORS

I'd like to thank all my clients from over the years. They've been a constant source of friendship and inspiration with their accomplishments both in fitness and in life. Their different movement restrictions, injuries, and questions have challenged me to continue learning, which has driven my professional development in directions I couldn't have chosen better myself.

The editorial and design staff at Callisto Media has been an amazing group of professionals and a pleasure to work with. Thank you for giving me the opportunity to help make this book a reality. —AS

ADAM SCHERSTEN is a certified personal trainer and top-tier trainer at the Equinox Printing House fitness club in Manhattan. An expert in bodyweight training and functional movement, he is the cofounder of First Move Wellness, a corporate wellness consultancy that teaches healthy biomechanics to prevent everyday pain and injury. To learn more, visit firstmovewellness.com.

CHRIS KLIMEK is a Washington, DC-based writer whose work regularly appears in *The Washington City Paper*, *The Washington Post*, *The Village Voice*, and on the NPR website. He is also a part-time boxing instructor.

CPSIA information can be obtained
at www.ICGtesting.com
Printed in the USA
BVOW05s1942170117
473739BV00001B/1/P

9 781623 157029